Janet Purchase

CHILDHOOD SYMPTOMS

CHILDHOOD SYMPTOMS

Every Parent's Guide to Childhood Illnesses

Edward R. Brace and
John P. Pacanowski, M.D., F.A.A.P.

A Stonesong Press Book

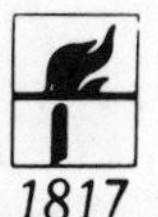

1817

HARPER & ROW, PUBLISHERS, New York
Cambridge, Philadelphia, San Francisco, London
Mexico City, São Paulo, Singapore, Sydney

Reprinted by permission of Harper & Row Publishers, Inc.

Grateful acknowledgment is made for permission to reprint an excerpt from *Pediatrics,* vol. 67, no. 5, May 1981, page 744. Copyright American Academy of Pediatrics, 1981.

 For information address Harper & Row, Publishers, Inc., 10 East 53rd Street, New York, N.Y. 10022. Published simultaneously in Canada by Fitzhenry & Whiteside Limited, Toronto.

FIRST EDITION

Designer: C. Linda Dingler

Library of Congress Cataloging in Publication Data

Brace, Edward R.
Childhood symptoms.

"A Stonesong Press book."
1. Pediatrics—Popular works. 2. Symptomatology.
I. Pacanowski, John P. II. Title. [DNLM: 1. Pediatrics
—handbooks. WS 39 B796p]
RJ61.B7888 1985 616.07'2 84-47974
ISBN 0-06-181098-3 10 9 8 7 6 5 4 3 2 1
ISBN 0-06-091152-2 (pbk.) 85 86 87 88 89 10 9 8 7 6 5 4 3 2 1

Contents

Important Telephone Numbers

Poison Control Center____________________________________

(See page 317 for Directory of Poison Control Centers)

Emergency Room____________________________________

Mobile Emergency Treatment Facility____________________

Police____

Fire Department______________________________________

Doctor____

Druggist____

Taxi____

Before You Call the Doctor

The following checklist will help you provide information to your child's doctor. Keep these points in mind when you call so the information you give the doctor is as thorough as possible.

1. In what way is the child sick or acting different?

2. How long has the condition been present?

3. What is the child's temperature and has it risen or declined recently?

4. Is the child taking any medicine? For how long?

5. Are there any allergies or reactions to medications?

6. Is the child in pain? Is there any swelling, bleeding, or discharge present?

7. Is there any difficulty breathing or swallowing? Has there been any vomiting or diarrhea?

8. Is there any bulging in the groin, abdomen, or scrotum?

9. Can the child's limbs be moved without pain?

10. Are there any rashes or other discoloration on the skin?

11. Are there any other symptoms or observations you think the doctor should know about?

12. Do you have any questions about the condition or the treatment of it?

Introduction

Parents are always deeply concerned when a child develops signs and symptoms of a potentially serious medical problem. What's wrong? What can it mean? Should I take the child to the doctor right away? *Childhood Symptoms* attempts to anticipate the types of questions a parent might like to ask the child's doctor and then provides clear answers to those questions.

The basic goal of *Childhood Symptoms* is to explain to parents and other concerned adults the significance of virtually all the signs and symptoms of diseases, disorders, and developmental problems that can affect infants, children, and adolescents. Entries are presented in alphabetical order to enhance quick access to essential information. In addition, an extensive system of cross-references, indicated by a term in SMALL CAPITAL LETTERS within the text of an entry or at the end of an entry, helps direct the reader from a specific symptom to those conditions in which that symptom may be important diagnostic evidence for the physician. The reader obtains a fully integrated discussion of specific symptoms and their most likely underlying cause.

In most cases a group of signs and symptoms will emerge that forms a pattern of a suspected illness. Only a qualified physician, with proper experience in identifying such patterns, can diagnose a suspected problem and offer the most effective modern treatment. A doctor often has to study the results of specific laboratory tests and other diagnostic procedures before confirming the diagnosis.

Readers must realize that the information contained in *Childhood Symptoms* should never be used as a substitute for professional medical care, or used to self-diagnose any specific problem a child may have. Rather, it is designed to provide helpful and general information that can be discussed openly with a child's physician. A parent or any daily caretaker who is knowledgeable about the signs and symptoms of childhood diseases is in a better position to aid the doctor in the main goal of returning an ill child to health as soon as possible.

—Edward R. Brace

CHILDHOOD ILLNESSES AND THEIR SIGNS AND SYMPTOMS

The information on pediatric symptoms and diseases contained in this book has been compiled from a variety of sources and is subject to differences of opinion and interpretation. This book is not intended to replace medical advice, and any questions on symptoms, general or specific, should be addressed to a physician.

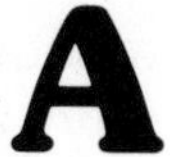

Abdominal bloating

The abdomen is that part of the body situated between the chest and the pelvis (lowest part of the trunk). The abdominal cavity contains organs such as the stomach, small intestine, large intestine or colon, liver, pancreas, spleen, kidneys, and bladder; in females it also contains the uterus and ovaries.

A newborn infant's abdomen normally appears larger than one would expect in relationship to other body parts. When a baby is lying down, the abdomen has a full, rounded appearance. As the youngster begins to stand and walk, the fullness becomes even more noticeable. At around the age of two years, as the abdominal muscles strengthen, the toddler's profile becomes flatter.

Some swelling or bloating may occur when a child is overfed or has swallowed an excessive amount of air. The problem is relieved when the child vomits or defecates. More persistent bloating may indicate that the child is not absorbing nutrients properly, a condition generally associated with poor weight gain. Chronic constipation may also cause the abdomen to look full and rounded. If persistent bloating is observed, medical attention should be sought.

In some instances swelling may indicate the presence of an abdominal mass. Generally this swelling is slow, progressive, and firm. But these tumors may be silent—that is, they cause no symptoms and a youngster does not complain, by whatever means available, whether verbally or just by exhibiting crankiness. For example, Wilms's tumor is one of the more common malignancies of childhood, usually occurring between the ages of six months to three years. The tumor affects the kidney. Once considered almost invariably fatal, Wilms's tumor can now often be successfully combatted by radiation therapy or chemotherapy as well as by surgical removal.

In the case of neuroblastomas—malignant growths that affect the sympathetic nervous system—at least one-third of children can be saved by surgery, chemotherapy, and radiation.

They can occur anywhere sympathetic nervous tissue is found, but they frequently appear as solid masses in the abdomen. These tumors are considered a disease of early childhood, occurring between birth and the age of six years.

An umbilical HERNIA involves a certain amount of localized protrusion.

Finally, there is abdominal bloating that can occur in the case of severe general infections or as a result of INTESTINAL OBSTRUCTION. Any abdominal distension that occurs very rapidly (say, in a matter of a few hours) and looks like an inflated balloon should alert a parent to the need for emergency treatment. In cases of intestinal obstruction, the child usually vomits profusely and is unable to retain even a small drink of water.

Remember that all young babies normally have protruding bellies that sometimes give them the appearance of a miniature Santa Claus. Parents should keep in mind that it is rapid abdominal distension that sounds the alarm. A prompt medical examination is in order whenever swelling of the abdomen exceeds the quantity or quality usually considered normal for their infants and toddlers. Other disorders not mentioned here combine to make abdominal bloating a serious sign that—except in an obvious instance of overeating or swallowing too much air—should never be ignored or downplayed.

Abdominal pain

One of the commonest complaints in childhood is that of abdominal pain. The abdominal cavity contains the stomach, small and large intestines, kidneys, bladder, liver, pancreas, spleen, and, in females, the reproductive organs. The first sign of an underlying problem affecting any of these organs may be abdominal pain. Although the causes are often minor—hunger, overeating, "gas," fatigue, or overexertion—a parent must be ever alert to the possibility of a significant medical condition.

The nature and apparent location of the discomfort are important diagnostic clues for the physician. For example, the pain may be sharp and highly localized in one area of the abdomen, or it may be experienced as a dull and poorly localized sensation. It may tend to come and go, in which case it is called cramping or intermittent, or be fairly constant.

The age of the child is another important factor in determining possible causes of abdominal pain. When a child is old enough to describe the nature of abdominal discomfort, it makes it much easier for the parents, and the physician, to determine what might be wrong—or at least to attempt to identify the most likely cause. In children too young to verbalize their discomfort, the diagnosis may be more difficult. Infants generally communicate their distress by crying. Distressed infants commonly cry in a way sensitive listeners can quickly distinguish from a feed-me cry.

Parents should note any associated signs or symptoms and describe them as accurately as they can. Is there vomiting or diarrhea? Has there been any fever? Are urinary symptoms present, such as burning or greater frequency? Is there a relationship to meals or feeding? When did the child last have a bowel movement? If the pain comes and goes, is there any apparent pattern in timing and intensity? Does anything seem to offer relief? Is the pain related to any signs of undue nervousness or agitation? If this is a recurrent bout, has there been a change in appetite or a loss of weight since the last episode? Is there a history of injury to the abdomen? The answers to such questions help your doctor assess the situation.

Acute APPENDICITIS is the most common emergency children experience that requires surgery. However, because the signs and symptoms resemble those of many other ailments, it may be difficult to diagnose accurately, and doctors usually perform laboratory tests in addition to taking a history and doing a physical examination. For example, a urinary-tract infection could mimic an attack of acute appendicitis. Appendicitis rarely occurs in infancy, and incidence decreases after age fourteen. Boys are stricken more often than girls. The pain, sometimes of a cramping nature, may start in the pit of the stomach and then shift to the lower right part of the abdomen. Frequently it begins around the navel and is experienced as a constant pain that increases in intensity before it moves to the lower right side.

As suggested, urinary-tract infections—as well as CYSTITIS (inflammation of the bladder) or KIDNEY INFECTIONS AND DISEASES—can cause abdominal pain. So can GASTROENTERITIS (inflammation of the stomach and intestines), INTESTINAL OBSTRUCTION, and PERITONITIS. Mild cases of gastroenteritis can often be traced to dietary causes or minor infections like the common cold, and they usually go away by themselves in a few days. Clearly, intestinal obstruction is a medical emergency, and infections or inflammations of the urinary tract should quickly be brought to medical attention. Frequently the sharpness and severity of the pain are clues to the seriousness of the condition.

Peptic ulcers, once believed to occur rarely in childhood, appear in fact to be more prevalent, although they are not too common. Older children tend to identify the pain as being in the pit of the stomach, while younger children place it around the navel.

Other cases of abdominal pain may be caused by certain abnormalities, such as Meckel's diverticulum (when a piece of embryonic tissue remains in the gut); INTUSSUSCEPTION (when a portion of intestine gets telescoped into another portion); and mesenteric adenitis (an appendicitis-mimicking disorder). Less serious causes of abdominal pain include infection by parasites such as roundworms, in which case the pain tends to be spasmodic and is often accompanied by nausea and vomiting.

Psychosomatic factors can also cause abdominal pain in children. A fear of school, social pressures, or anxiety can cause pain that is experienced as quite real. Children need to have this pain recognized and dealt with either by reassurance and supportive measures or through professional consultation.

Fortunately most cases of abdominal pain in children are not serious. However, if the pain comes on suddenly or persists for more than an hour or two, seek a physician's help, especially if the pain is accompanied by vomiting. Do *not* give the child solid foods until advised to do so by the child's doctor. If the child is thirsty, he or she may be given small sips of water or other cool drinks with the doctor's permission. But if these fluids are not retained, call the doctor again. Above all, children with acute abdominal pain should never be given a laxative or cathartic. In certain conditions, including appendicitis, such medicines could cause intestinal damage and further pain.

Acne

Acne vulgaris—the Latin name for common acne—involves an inflammation of the sebaceous glands that produces pimples, the small, red swellings that often exude pus. Acne usually affects glands in facial skin as well as on the chest and back.

Although acne sometimes afflicts preteenagers and adults, the skin disorder is most common during adolescence. This is the time that androgenic hormones are first secreted into the bloodstream. Unfortunately it is also the time at which most young people take a new and sudden interest in their body image, how they look, and whether they are attractive.

There is no good time to have acne. Well-meaning parents —and even well-meaning doctors—can reassure adolescents all they want that having acne is part of growing up and that it will not last forever. Adolescents know better. The fact of the matter is that except for the mildest Grade I acne, the lesions *are* unslightly and disfiguring, and to an adolescent, when waiting for the next school dance seems like forever, the thought of waiting two, four, or six years for this condition to clear is intolerable.

Fortunately, some promising new treatments exist in which benzoyl peroxide is applied for progressively longer periods to promote drying and peeling. Some people, however, react adversely to the chemical, as noted below.

Androgenic hormones cause increased activity of the sebaceous glands, the oil glands, of the skin. Sebum, the sticky substance produced by these glands, sometimes fills and stretches the skin pores. The result: blackheads. These blackheads block the pores, preventing natural skin oils from reaching the surface. As these blocked oils collect beneath the outside surface of the skin, they form tiny cysts. When the cysts break, harmful bacteria can cross the skin's "protective barrier," causing inflammation and infection.

As affected adolescents know, there is acne and there is acne. The so-called Pillsbury Classifications cover four degrees of severity. Grade I is a relatively mild condition in which there are blackheads and whiteheads and a vaguely pimply appearance, but no serious interference with the adolescent's appearance—except possibly in his or her own estimation. This type of acne responds to simple home remedies.

Grade II features more and more enlarged whiteheads that are deeply impacted and may cover the whole face. In Grade III there are enlarged and swollen, pus-filled eruptions in addition to blackheads and whiteheads. In Grade IV acne the sufferer's face is likely to be covered with raw-looking, purple-colored, large cysts in addition to the smaller lesions. This is truly disfiguring and deeply traumatic to the affected teenager.

Regardless of the grade of acne, the pimples that form around pore openings should not be squeezed; this may spread any infection that is present or cause a second infection from harmful bacteria on the skin surface or underneath fingernails.

Treatment depends on severity. Since it is seldom an easy task for sufferers or their parents to determine if both inflammation and infection are present, it is best to consult a doctor or perhaps a dermatologist (a skin specialist), who is apt to be aware of the newest acne treatments, such as isotretinoin, available under the trade name Accutane, a prescription drug that can be taken for extremely severe cystic acne.

In simple cases, it may be sufficient simply to wash the affected areas with soap and water and apply drying solutions. Antibacterial soaps seem to offer no added benefit. Several non-prescription products may help. Among the most useful are those that contain benzoyl peroxide, a chemical that helps dry the skin and remove excess oil. But use of these products should be discontinued at the first sign of excessive itching, burning, redness, or extreme drying of the skin.

Addiction, warning signs of

It seems a bit bizarre for parents with a martini in one hand and a cigarette in the other to approach their preteen or teenage child and announce, "Don't you ever fool around with marijuana!"

Adolescents frequently experiment with drugs because of peer pressure, general rebelliousness, or at times, particularly with alcohol, because they think this is grown-up behavior. Parental intervention just might exacerbate the situation.

Substance abuse to the point of addiction, however, necessitates that a professional counselor enter the scene. Dependency might be suggested by school truancy and lowered academic performance, seeming lack of initiative, confusion, bizarre behavior, and inappropriate spending of money. Perhaps of more significance—since any adolescent might engage in such behaviors from time to time—are noticeable physical signs, such as unusual nasal congestion, changes in appetite, glassy eyes, or marked changes in behavior, such as being hyper (overactive) or very fatigued.

Direct confrontation doesn't work. Parents should check with an appropriately trained professional—a physician or counselor, a social agency or drug counseling center, or a member of the clergy—who is experienced in this field.

Adenoids

See TONSILS AND ADENOIDS.

Aggressive behavior

A form of behavior in which a child displays a strong tendency toward fighting, instigating disorder, and infringing on the rights of others.

Many theories have been advanced to explain how a pattern of aggressive behavior may develop—for example, bad behavior may lead to punishment may lead to anger and aggressive feelings may lead to bad behavior. Violence on television and aggressive "models" such as a parent or older sibling have also been suggested as causes.

Perhaps of most importance to the concerned parent is the realization that behavior that may be entirely appropriate at the age of two may be totally inappropriate at the age of eight or twelve. When the child is showing behavior that is out of the ordinary for same-age peers or for certain social situations, parents shouldn't block it from their minds in the mistaken belief that it is just a phase. Or, in the event of a teacher complaining that the child is unruly or provocative, parents should try not to fall into the trap of believing that their child is all right and it's the outsiders who are wrong.

If a careful and honest review of the home atmosphere fails to reveal causes or contributors that are easily remedied, the situation should be discussed at once with the child's pediatrician or a professional counselor. The sooner a repair process begins, the better the likelihood of a successful outcome.

Alcohol usage

See ADDICTION, WARNING SIGNS OF.

Allergic rhinitis

See HAY FEVER.

Allergy

Any condition in which a person becomes unusually sensitive to some substance(s) or physical agent(s). Nothing happens during the first encounter. In fact, it may take several years for an individual to become "sensitized" to the point at which an allergy develops. But once this sensitization occurs, the now-allergic person suffers a typical reaction every time he or she encounters the offending material.

The substance that triggers an allergic reaction in a sensitized person is called an allergen. It may be pollen, animal hair or dander, fur, house dust, an insect bite or sting, certain foods, some antibiotics (especially penicillin), and many others. An allergic reaction may also be caused or heightened by emotional states or by cold, heat, and sunlight. Most allergies are more annoying than serious, although in rare instances a severe allergic reaction called ANAPHYLACTIC SHOCK can be a direct threat to life.

Children as well as adults are subject to a wide variety of allergies. Sometimes allergies have a hereditary basis, although a specific allergy is not always passed on to children. The most common sites for allergic reactions are the skin, the air passages to the lungs, the nose, and the digestive tract. Disorders include ECZEMA and HIVES, allergic BRONCHITIS and ASTHMA, HAY FEVER, and some conditions affecting the intestinal tract.

An allergic reaction involves the breakdown of the immune mechanisms, the body's normal defense against disease. The body normally responds to bacterial infection by producing protective substances called antibodies, which are released into the bloodstream to attack the bacteria. In many cases the protective substances remain in the body for years, providing partial or total immunity to further attacks of the same disease. The body of an allergic person treats certain substances—for example, pollen, feathers, or shellfish—as if they were disease-causing invaders such as bacteria. The basic mechanism of the allergic reaction is the same; it is the site that is affected that determines the specific outcome. For example, allergens that meet allergic antibodies in the skin cause hives.

Histamine plays a special role in allergies as do many other naturally occurring body chemicals. A normal body substance, histamine is concentrated largely in those tissues that have direct or indirect contact with the air: the skin, the lining of the nose, and the lungs. In the case of injury or infection, certain amounts of histamine are normally released into affected tissues. Histamine causes a dilation, or opening, of the smaller blood vessels at the site of an injury and contributes to the so-called inflammatory response, which is a natural feature of the healing process. This response allows the escape of some plasma (the clear fluid portion of blood) through the walls of tiny blood vessels and into surrounding tissues, which results in the swelling that accompanies many injuries and infections.

Often it is the sudden release of histamine and other substances that is responsible for the signs and symptoms of an allergic reaction. In a sensitized individual, when an invading allergen comes in contact with a body cell to which an allergic antibody is attached, it causes the dramatic response known as the allergic reaction. These compounds are released from such cells in greater amounts than would be normal, that is, normal in the case of injury or infection. Depending on the site of the allergic reaction, this can cause swelling, redness, and itching of the skin, sometimes with the formation of wheals or bumps; inflammation and swelling of the mucous membranes of the nose, causing nasal congestion or a stuffy nose; constriction or spasm of the alveoli, the small air passages in the lungs; and increased activity of the digestive tract.

Relief can frequently be obtained by taking antihistamines —"anti" meaning that they act to neutralize or inhibit the action of histamine. For relatively minor problems, sufferers may use an antihistamine that is available without prescription. More powerful antihistamines and other medications for more severe allergic reactions can be prescribed by a physician. Since the age of the child and the exact nature of the allergy are important factors to consider, parents may want to check with the child's doctor and also carefully read the "children's dose" information accompanying any nonprescription preparation.

Alopecia

See HAIR, LOSS AND THINNING.

Amebic dysentery

A disease caused by the infectious single-cell organisms called *Entamoeba histolytica,* in which there is inflammation of the mucous membranes of the intestine, abdominal pain, and severe diarrhea with blood or mucus typically being passed in loose, watery stools. Children are by no means spared such infections, which occur worldwide—although they are more common in tropical countries or underdeveloped areas where standards of hygiene are inadequate.

The disease is spread from human feces or stools that contain a cystic form of the ameba. In this form, the ameba cells build a protective wall around themselves. If they are swallowed in food or water that's contaminated with them, they eventually shed this wall in the human intestines, where they begin to multiply and cause dysentery.

At first the inflammation of the walls of the colon (large intestine) causes the child to experience painful passage of stools, which are often stained with mucus and blood. The infection may cause erosion or ulceration of the intestinal wall, leading to abscesses.

For diagnostic purposes, microscopic examination must be made of the child's stool. It's especially important for the doctor to distinguish the disease from BACILLARY DYSENTERY. Treatment depends on severity. Bed rest and a bland diet will be necessary until all signs of infection have disappeared. In many cases drugs such as emetine or metronidazole may be prescribed. It is important to obtain appropriate medical care because, left untreated, the infection can enter the bloodstream and be carried to the liver, lungs, or, more rarely, to the pericardium (the sac that surrounds the heart).

Anal fissures

A tear or cracking of the lining around the anus (the external opening at the end of the digestive tract). The tear usually results from the child having a large, hard bowel movement or straining excessively when going to the bathroom. On occasion it may occur after bouts of diarrhea, when unusually runny stools have irritated the area.

Generally speaking, the condition should be suspected when blood, usually bright red in color, is noted on the outside of the bowel movement or, in toilet-trained youngsters, on toilet paper used for wiping. The amount of blood is usually small—less than a teaspoon—and the bleeding generally stops spontaneously. If the bleeding is larger in volume or if the blood is mixed with the bowel movement, there may be a problem higher in the intestine. Medical attention should be sought at once.

A parent can usually determine if an anal fissure is present. If the child or infant's buttocks are spread wide enough, the fissure will appear as a raw-looking crack around the rim of the anal opening itself, with normal tissue on either side.

Treatment can be both direct and indirect; usually a combination works best. The fissure itself should be thoroughly cleansed with mild soap and water after each bowel movement. Sitz baths are especially useful. The older child can soak his or her bottom in slightly warm, but not hot, water for twenty minutes two or three times a day. The infant or toddler who must be supported, of course, has to be held so that the water soaks the anal area. At times special creams may be helpful, but parents should first discuss this with the child's physician. Inserting glycerin suppositories lubricates the area and eases passage of stools in children who are straining.

When hard bowel movements seem to be causing the difficulty, a change in diet may help, since more roughage is needed. Bran cereals or commercially available stool softeners hold more water in the stool, making it softer and easier to pass. If the problem persists, a physician should be consulted.

Anal itching

Anal itching, technically called pruritus ani, can be caused by moist or irritating underwear or diapers. Sometimes it is caused by some other inflammation or is the result of anal fissure or worm infestation.

Treatment of anal itching must be directed at the underlying cause. But relief of symptoms can be obtained by carefully washing with mild soap and then drying the area with a soft cloth or tissue. The application of a fine powder can help reduce any moisture.

See also: ANAL FISSURES, PINWORMS.

Anaphylactic shock

The most serious form of allergic reaction. Under ALLERGY the reader will find a description of how someone becomes sensitized to a foreign substance. In anaphylactic shock, also known as anaphylactic reaction, the sensitized person experiences a sudden and explosive reaction when confronted by the allergen—perhaps injection of a drug such as penicillin or use of a diagnostic agent such as X-ray contrast medium, or the sting of a bee or wasp, or eating some seemingly innocuous food such as strawberries or shellfish. A typical reaction includes severe interference with breathing (caused by spasm of the tiny air passages in the lungs or swelling of the throat); hypotension (a sudden drop in blood pressure); and, in some occasions, convulsions and loss of consciousness. In some instances death can occur.

Emergency treatment of anaphylactic shock includes injection of epinephrine (adrenaline) and administration of an antihistamine (either by injection or, if the child is able to swallow, by mouth). Sometimes it may also be necessary to add to blood volume by intravenously administering a special salt solution.

Regardless of the availability of emergency medical treatment, the best precaution is avoiding any substance to which the child is known to be sensitive. In the case of wasps and bees, stay away from areas where they are known to nest and flourish. Sensitive children should avoid wearing bright or pastel-color clothing when outdoors, and parents should consider avoiding colognes or scented lotions that could attract insects.

Not all anaphylactic reactions are life threatening. But to the child suddenly stricken by difficult breathing and the cold, clammy kind of faintness that accompanies a sudden drop in blood pressure, the distinction is very fine indeed. Therefore, it is helpful to have some tablet-form antihistamines at hand for emergency use. Large doses of over-the-counter ones may do the trick, or your child's pediatrician may prescribe a stronger antihistamine.

A kit containing epinephrine and a chewable antihistamine is available by prescription and should *always* be kept on hand if you have a child who has a history of one of the more severe reactions.

Also, parents can discuss desensitization with their child's doctor, if the child has a history of severe reactions to bee stings and other allergens.

See also: ALLERGY.

Anemia

A condition in which the red blood cells are reduced below a certain volume or do not have adequate oxygen-carrying capacity.

The former situation is measured by what doctors call the hematocrit; the latter, by what's termed the hemoglobin percent. Normal values have been established by checking large numbers of healthy individuals over a long period of time. These normal values change according to the age of the child. For example, at birth an infant may show a hematocrit of between 50 and 70 percent and a hemoglobin of around 16 to 18 grams per 100 cubic centimeters (cc). Because red-cell production normally falls off right after birth, both these measurements will fall to their lowest points between the first eight to twelve weeks of life (approximately 35 percent and about 11 to 12 grams per 100 cc, respectively). This falloff is normal and requires no therapy. Later on children usually show a certain range that averages out to the following:

	Hematocrit, percent	Hemoglobin, percent
6 months–6 years	37	12
7 years–12 years	38	13
Over 12 years		
females	42	14
males	47	16

There are many causes for anemia. In nutritional anemia, the most common form, there is simply not enough iron available for blood-cell formation. Sometimes infants who consume large quantities of milk and very little else show this kind of anemia. Loss of blood, for whatever reason, may be a cause, as can some infections and certain chronic illnesses. There are also congenital or familial anemias, such as sickle cell anemia, which result from defective formation of red blood cells.

Children who are anemic appear pale, listless, and inattentive. A severely anemic child tires easily or perhaps becomes short of breath when active. Excessive thirst may be a problem, and adolescents sometimes chew or suck on ice cubes. However, it's frequently the case that no significant symptoms or signs are noted by parents, and only blood tests will show the anemia.

Both the diagnosis and the treatment of an anemic condition should be carried out by a qualified physician. Sometimes a specialty consultant, a hematologist, is consulted. If a child is listless, parents should not attempt to treat the condition by giving iron supplements. First of all, if the child is not really anemic, the iron is of no value. Second, and more important, large amounts can be dangerous to children. Too much iron can cause gastrointestinal upset, staining of teeth, and, if really excessive, siderosis (a disease that results from excess iron circulating in the blood).

Angioma

See HEMANGIOMA.

Animal bites

Any breaks in the skin caused by an animal's teeth, as well as any scratches that come in contact with an animal's saliva, require prompt attention. The area should be cleansed thoroughly with soap and water and then flushed with peroxide. If the wound is large or there is significant bleeding, the child should be taken to an emergency medical facility. In some localities any animal bite must be reported to the police.

In conjunction with the area's health department, the physician will decide what, if any, additional therapy may be needed. A decision to immunize the child with RABIES vaccine depends on a number of factors, including the prevalence or absence of rabies in local animals.

The child's general immunization history should be reviewed. Children who have not had a TETANUS booster within the past five years should get one. The wound must be observed carefully for redness, swelling, or drainage, indicating the presence of an infection that would require antibiotic treatment. Frequently antibiotics are started at the time of initial therapy so that infections are prevented.

Any cat or dog that inflicts a bite must be captured and examined by a veterinarian. The animal should be observed for ten days. If it develops signs of illness, the animal must be destroyed so the brain can be examined for signs of rabies. Unprovoked attacks—that is, when the animal was not teased, hurt, or otherwise annoyed—cause greater concern that the animal may be rabid. Even though many pet animals are immunized, it is possible that the vaccine was ineffective or that it actually produced the disease. So the rules for confinement and observation should always be followed.

Among wild animals, skunks and bats have the highest incidence of rabies infection. Other wild, meat-eating animals, including raccoons, also have a greater chance of becoming infected. Smaller animals—rats, rabbits, squirrels, hamsters, gerbils —seldom get the disease; but to be safe, one should check with a physician or a local emergency room whenever an animal bite occurs.

Ankle pain

A complaint of discomfort in the ankle joint is usually a sign that the child has twisted the ankle when falling or jumping. Frequently there is a mild to moderate amount of swelling and the pain is greatest when the child tries to walk. Ankle-area ligaments (fibers that connect bone to bone) are stretched—sometimes torn—and there may be a kind of "pocket" of fluid where blood or blood plasma has accumulated. If there is considerable swelling and very severe pain, an X ray is needed to determine whether one of the lower leg bones or the ankle itself may have been fractured.

An extremely forceful sprain may completely tear the ligaments along either side of the ankle. This means the joint will be unstable, and special treatment, usually directed by an orthopedic surgeon, will be needed.

In the case of a simple ankle sprain, treatment consists of elevating the leg and foot, applying ice packs, and rest. Walking before the swelling has subsided only prolongs the repair process by aggravating the original injury, tearing more fibers, and further weakening the joint. If the sprain is unusually severe, a physician may apply a short walking cast even though no fracture is present.

Other causes of ankle pain include improper footwear or structural deformities of the feet such as fallen arches; the presence of a more generalized disease such as RHEUMATIC FEVER or JUVENILE RHEUMATOID ARTHRITIS; or, when there is no history of injury, a possible bone cyst or tumor. X-ray examination and medical attention will be required.

Anorexia

Diminished appetite. Unlike the serious condition of ANOREXIA NERVOSA, simple diminished appetite often accompanies the onset of fever or the development of some physical illness or emotional upset. Once the underlying cause of appetite suppression is dealt with, the child's eating habits will return to normal.

Anorexia nervosa

An abnormal and prolonged suppression of appetite related to mental, emotional, or some yet unknown metabolic illness and characterized by excessive weight loss, often resulting in an emaciated, almost skeletal appearance. The condition mainly affects preadolescent and adolescent girls and seems to be connected with body image and an irrational fear of being overweight. Sufferers seem to be totally preoccupied with weight, even if they become grossly underweight and emaciated. The condition is not associated with any underlying physical disease known at this time.

While these individuals frequently seem never to eat, they do not always lose their appetites altogether. Indeed, many girls alternate anorexia nervosa with periods of bulimia, an excessively abnormal increase in appetite. They may go on eating binges and consume huge quantities of favorite foods such as chocolate sundaes before they then force themselves to vomit.

Their preoccupation with food often leads them to collect diets and recipes, prepare large and fancy dinners for other people, and sometimes hoard and waste food.

Emotionally they are often quite depressed. Behaviorally they often become highly manipulative, managing to "get what they want" out of concerned family members or professionals by using eating as a bargaining tool.

Physically, the child with anorexia nervosa may show abnormal patterns of growth in body and facial hair, low blood pressure and low body temperature, and menstrual difficulties, including amenorrhea (having no menstrual periods).

Home treatment is definitely not recommended. When there has been very significant weight loss, hospitalization may be required, initially with the possibility of tube feeding or "forced feeding." Drastic as the measures may seem, they may become necessary just so that a minimal weight and basic physical health are maintained. Gradually, independence and more mature behavior are encouraged.

Frequently family therapy with a counselor skilled in dealing with anorexia nervosa patients and their parents may be advisable. Underlying causes seem to be multiple and complicated, and recovery can be slow. Therefore, the adage "the sooner the better" applies when it comes to treatment; otherwise the disorder can lead to very severe nutritional deficiencies and even death by starvation or related complications.

Anxiety

See FEARS.

Appendicitis

An inflammation of the appendix, that small wormlike tube, closed at its free end, that juts down from the cecum, a kind of pouch that forms the beginning portion of the large intestine.

The appendix is about the length and half the diameter of an adult's little finger, and it usually hangs freely within the abdominal cavity. The interior of the appendix is very narrow. Sometimes hard pieces of waste matter or foreign bodies become trapped within it, causing an obstruction leading to severe inflammation. It can also become inflamed as the result of a general infection or when an abscess spreads from a nearby area.

Children of any age can be stricken with appendicitis, although adolescents seem to be at greater risk. It has been estimated that in the United States 4 out of every 1000 children undergo an appendectomy each year. For unknown reasons the peak incidence of appendicitis occurs in autumn and spring, and males are affected more often than females.

Symptoms and signs vary from one individual to the next. Usually pain begins in the middle of the abdomen or the "pit of the stomach" and later moves to the lower right side of the abdomen. Nausea and vomiting generally develop early on. Because the peritoneum is irritated, movement causes pain; coughing hurts and a child may walk bent over. If the appendix has ruptured, a child's temperature may reach 104°F (40°C).

If the slightest suspicion exists that the child's tummy ache could be appendicitis, *never* give a laxative. This could hasten rupture. The first rule is: call a physician at the very first hint that the child may have appendicitis. Delay could also result in a rupture, which can be life threatening, even in today's era of powerful antibiotics.

In an acute attack of appendicitis, the blood supply to the

appendix is interrupted. This, in turn, can lead to gangrene, that is, death of part of its tissues. If the infected appendix ruptures, PERITONITIS may develop. Treatment of acute appendicitis involves surgical removal of the inflamed appendix. It is a relatively simple operation that requires only a short stay in the hospital.

Appetite changes

An almost constant concern to most parents is what and how much their children eat. Books on nutrition are widely available, and many of them offer some reasonable guidelines.

Normal eating patterns vary during a child's growing years. During the first year of life, an infant gains weight and grows in length at a pace never to be achieved again. By one year the birth weight is tripled and the baby has grown about ten inches. Because of the demands posed by this growth, a baby eats what seems like an incredible amount of milk and solids. At the end of the first year, however, the growth rate slows noticeably and does not pick up much until adolescence.

In the preschool years a child's weight gain is about five pounds a year; the increase in height, about two and one-half inches. During this time children's appetites decrease considerably. A demand for fluids remains, but a toddler may go for extended periods of time—even for a few days—without wanting much in the way of solids. This can be frustrating to parents, and if they're not careful they may unwittingly contribute to future feeding difficulties for the child. Undue concern on the parents' part can force children to become obstinate about eating; then a vicious cycle develops.

While nutritious, balanced foods should be offered on a regular basis, do not always demand that they be eaten. Similarly, junk foods, excessive sweets, and carbonated beverages should be avoided as a routine—but an occasional treat will be greeted happily and possibly also convince a child that meals are okay, too.

Parents who get upset when their children don't eat may benefit from an interesting experiment. Fill your plate with the following: a one-pound patty of ground beef, four cups of french fries, and three cups of some vegetable you're not particularly fond of. Then fill a one-quart pitcher three-quarters full of milk.

Now, despite your busy afternoon and the fact that you may not feel very hungry, sit down and quietly eat this dinner! Since you weigh about three or four times what your child does, these portions may equal what you put on a child's plate. The moral of the story: be careful to serve children portions they can handle. Also, listen to what your children tell you. They just may know what is good for them. Remember the old "ideal breakfast" with eggs and two or three strips of bacon? These foods happen to contain high amounts of cholesterol, saturated fat, and salt, not to mention potentially dangerous preservatives in most bacon.

Finally, keep in mind that meals should be a pleasant, restful time with an air of ease; a time to take care of self and a time to talk about the day's activities. Any demand for another kind of performance—that is, eating—makes the period stressful for the child.

Remember, too, that when children reach their next period of growth spurt—adolescence—they will probably munch their way through everything that is not nailed to the floor.

In general, parents should not worry about changes in appetite unless the child shows noticeable weight loss, fever, marked irritability, or gastrointestinal symptoms, any of which may signal a possible disease state.

Compare FEEDING PATTERN CHANGES.

Arches

See FLAT FEET.

Arrhythmia

Any abnormal rhythm or disturbance of the natural or expected rhythm, especially of the heartbeat. Some children have a harmless condition known as sinus arrthythmia, in which the pulse rate increases when they breathe in and decreases when they breathe out. It is rarely associated with other symptoms, although in some instances the change in rate is so pronounced that the rhythm seems to be quite irregular.

See also: HEART RATE, HEART MURMURS, PALPITATION.

Arthritis

A disease of a bony joint in which there is both swelling and pain. Occasionally it is a localized or isolated problem that may stem from infection by invading bacteria. However, most commonly the swelling and pain occur because of some systemic disease such as JUVENILE RHEUMATOID ARTHRITIS, RHEUMATIC FEVER, or LUPUS ERYTHEMATOSUS.

See also: JOINT PAIN.

Artificial respiration

See CARDIOPULMONARY RESUSCITATION.

Ascariasis

Infestation of the intestines with a specific type of parasitic roundworm called *Ascaris lumbricoides.* Children under the age of about twelve years are most likely to be affected, and the possible complication of intestinal obstruction is noted mostly in children under the age of six.

The infective eggs of these worms develop in soil. Very young children may take them in simply by putting dirt into their mouths. Older children may become infected as a result of putting contaminated fingers or toys into their mouths.

The eggs hatch inside the intestines and then may be circulated to the lungs and to the epiglottis (a lidlike structure that covers the larynx or voice box). Here they may be reswallowed and go back to the intestine as adult worms, so more eggs are laid and the cycle continues.

Often the child shows no symptoms and the condition goes unnoticed unless a parent happens to find a worm in the child's bowel movement. If symptoms do occur, children usually show intermittent pain in the abdomen or in the "pit of the stomach"; loss of appetite and perhaps some weight loss; and, if the worms pass through the lungs, a kind of pneumonia or perhaps asthma-like episodes.

Diagnosis is made by identifying a worm that is passed in

the child's stools or by looking for the eggs in a stool specimen with a microscope. Treatment will typically involve the use of antiparasitic drugs such as piperazine citrate, pyrantel pamoate, or mebendazole.

Asthma

A disorder that affects the small air passages of the lungs, constricting them so that breathing becomes difficult and very labored. In order to get enough air affected children may have to sit upright and forcibly lift and drop their shoulders. Typically there are sudden attacks of breathlessness and wheezing, and a bout leaves the sufferer exhausted.

Many factors can cause or contribute to asthma. Three major ones are ALLERGY (including a family history of allergies such as hay fever, eczema, and asthma itself), emotional stress, and infection. Asthma can start at any age, but when it begins early in childhood, it is most commonly caused by an allergy.

Inhaled pollen, dust, molds, and animal danders as well as certain foods are common offenders. When the foreign substance causes a sudden release of histamine and other compounds from the cells of tissues in the lungs' smaller air passages, the mucous membranes swell and the muscles tighten, causing the constriction. In addition, thick and sticky mucus is secreted, further blocking air passages and making breathing even more difficult.

Allergic asthma can be seasonal (for example, a reaction to high pollen count) or it may occur at any time of the year. In most cases asthmatic attacks occur in isolated episodes, although they can last from a few minutes or hours to up to several days in chronic patients. In severe cases asthmatic attacks can be extremely frightening to both the children and their parents. The victim often believes that suffocation is taking place, and this fear only serves to intensify the attack. Therefore, it is essential that concerned parents shield their own anxiety from the child as much as possible—there's enough dread already!

Asthmatic attacks often occur at night. When a bout starts, try to stay as calm as possible. Don't panic. Sit near the child or on the edge of the bed and speak softly and reassuringly during the attack. If the child has had previous attacks and medications have been prescribed, give them exactly as directed. Cool, clear liquids may be given to help loosen the mucous secretions. Watch carefully for the progress of the attack. If the respiratory rate continues to increase or the breathing seems to be getting more labored after a reasonable period of time—perhaps an hour—the child should be taken to an emergency room for inhalation or other kinds of therapy. When there have been no previous episodes of wheezing, the child should be taken to a physician so that an accurate diagnosis can be made and treatment begun.

Even in the presence of a known allergen (the substance that triggers an allergic reaction), the emotional factor may be more obvious in children than in adults. In children susceptible to asthma, tension at home or constant parental arguing can play a key role in the frequency and severity of attacks.

Various drugs exist that can be prescribed by the child's physician to lessen the frequency and severity of the attacks. The doctor can also help by suggesting ways to alleviate tensions or family problems that may be contributing to the asthma.

Bronchodilators (medicines that dilate the bronchial tubes) and some antiasthmatic drugs are available without a doctor's prescription. However, these over-the-counter products should *never* be used unless a physician has actually made the diagnosis of asthma. Also, if such products seem to cause a worsening of the child's condition, medical help should be sought at once.

Both parents and an asthmatic child can take some reassurance from the fact that children often—but not always—outgrow their asthma, although sometimes some other allergic condition, such as hay fever, remains as part of the original sensitivity. In some chronic sufferers the outlook is not so promising, and a doctor should be consulted at regular intervals for the monitoring and treatment of the disorder.

Athlete's foot

A fungus infection of the foot, characterized by redness, itching, cracking and scaling of the skin, especially between the toes, and sometimes by the formation of watery blisters. The condition is not common in younger children, but it may become a recurring problem for preadolescent and adolescent youths who engage in sports programs or are otherwise in settings where showers and other facilities are shared by many pairs of youthful bare feet, such as at summer camp.

Children's feet often sweat excessively, and the moisture may cause irritation. Also, allergic reactions to dyes and glues used in footwear may cause symptoms similar to athlete's foot. Microscopic examination of a scraping from the skin will settle the question of diagnosis.

Managing the disease requires some close attention to the frequent washing of clothes, bed linens, and towels. Children should be instructed to be sure to dry between their toes after bathing, and they should avoid footwear that prevents an adequate amount of air from reaching the feet.

Mild infections can be treated by dusting the feet with an absorbent antifungal powder such as zinc undecylenate. In more persistent infections, a physician may prescribe applications of clotrimazole or miconazole nitrate.

Attention deficit disorders

Formerly tagged as having minimal brain dysfunction (MBD), children or adolescents with attention deficit disorders generally have perfectly normal or even above-normal intelligence. But some neurological imbalance contributes to their difficulty in maintaining alertness or attention to some task at hand. They may also experience problems with IMPULSIVITY and HYPERACTIVITY.

The combined efforts of parents, medical and psychological professionals, and the child's teacher are necessary to deal with this condition. Parents who suspect an attention deficit disorder in their child should promptly seek professional assessment.

Attention span, short

The child's inability to maintain concentration on some given task or thought. It may be a feature in LEARNING DISABILITY and is a typical symptom of the ATTENTION DEFICIT DISORDERS.

As most parents have already observed, the very young toddler tends to move quickly from one activity to another. By the time youngsters are ready for school, they can usually work through the beginning, middle, and end of an activity and the impulsivity characteristic of the toddler stage has been curbed by many socialization influences.

Children with short attention spans most often bring to school a set of behaviors that is really characteristic of an earlier stage of development. They may be seen as "misbehaving" and be disciplined because of it; since they really cannot control their efforts, such children tend to become angry and thus even less amenable to learning.

Psychological testing may be helpful in defining the problem and suggesting methods of coping with it. In some instances medication may improve the attention span by lessening hyperactivity. Professional help is required and should be sought early to prevent the child from growing up with a poor self-image and from being regarded as a troublemaker.

Autism

A severe disorder of communication and behavior, sometimes called infantile autism or infantile psychosis, typically noted during a child's first few months of life and invariably present by the time the child who has this disorder reaches the age of three years. The disorder is characterized by a profound and almost total withdrawal from all human contact—even an avoidance of eye contact. Autistic children repel attempts at cuddling or play. They may engage in bizarre activities, such as banging their heads against walls. They often form attachments to inanimate objects and show an obsessive need for sameness or ritual. If their routines are disrupted, they may throw violent temper tantrums. There is often considerable mental retardation, but even when this is not the case, the development of speech is seriously delayed or virtually absent.

The cause of infantile autism is unknown. There is absolutely no evidence to suggest that the condition is associated with parental rejection, as was once believed.

If communicative speech does not develop by about the age of five, the outlook is generally poor. Psychological tests are difficult to administer, but, in skillful hands, can help define the limits of expected development. If the general intelligence is not severely impaired, a normal school education may be possible for those children who are amenable to behavior-therapy techniques and whose parents are patient enough to apply them after professional guidance.

Generally speaking, no specific treatment exists, although tranquilizers are sometimes prescribed to relieve symptoms such as screaming attacks and extreme hyperactivity. In severe forms of autism it may be necessary to institutionalize the child.

B

Bacillary dysentery

An acute infectious disease, also known as shigellosis, of the large intestine caused by a particular type of bacteria called *Shigella*. The disease-causing microorganisms are transmitted in the stools of infected persons and may be picked up and carried by flies or through the handling of contaminated foods or other objects. As one might expect, the disease is most common in areas of overcrowding, where sanitation is poor.

The sufferer typically experiences a profuse diarrhea in which the frequent stools are watery and streaked with mucus and blood. Other symptoms and signs include abdominal cramps, spasmodic contractions of the muscle ring that surrounds the anus, general weakness, and fever. Children with bacillary dysentery may run extremely high fevers and experience convulsions. Diagnosis is made by identifying the bacteria in a stool sample. Often an examination of the bottommost section of the large intestine will show certain destructive changes in the intestinal wall that rarely occur in amebic dysentery.

The incubation period from infection to symptoms is usually two to three days. The severity of the disease will depend upon the exact species of bacteria and the sufferer's general health. If a child is suffering from malnutrition or is already run down because of another disease, the death rate can be high. However, in the majority of uncomplicated cases, the disease will run its course and spontaneously clear up in about a week. More severe infections may last for six weeks or more.

Bed rest and fluid replacement, either by mouth or administered through a vein, form the best therapeutic approach. Fluid replacement is necessary because the infection causes serious loss of essential body fluids and the elements they contain, particularly salt. In more severe cases a physician may want to prescribe antibiotics.

Back pain

The spine is actually a series of joints similar to those elsewhere in the human body, even though most people don't regard the "backbone" as such. Alongside this system of bones and ligaments (fibers that connect bone to bone) are elongated muscle masses that allow movement and also provide stability. An injury to the bone or ligaments, or a severe pull on these back muscles, will cause a spasm. The spasm acts to prevent further movement by the simple mechanism of causing pain. Children may twist their backs while playing, cause strain by lifting objects too heavy for them, or sustain a direct injury to the back, perhaps by falling. The painful discomfort caused is usually aggravated by movement and may be partially relieved by having the child lie on a firm, flat surface.

Treatment of back strains generally consists of rest, taking aspirin as often as the directions say is acceptable for children, and the use of moist heat—just dampen towels in hot water. Sleeping on a rug or pad on the floor may also help. Rest should be continued until walking or engaging in other movements does not cause pain. If these measures don't bring a pattern of steady improvement, medical evaluation is necessary to determine if a more serious problem exists.

Although unusual in childhood but occasionally seen in late adolescence, back discomfort associated with pain in the buttocks or the legs may occur because of a protruding intervertebral disk ("slipped disk"), and special X rays are required to make this diagnosis.

When the pain strikes suddenly and there is no known injury, several possibilities must be considered. Back discomfort can occur in flu-type illnesses; it's usually connected with a generalized achy feeling. In the case of KIDNEY INFECTIONS, the pain is usually off to one side or the other rather than in the center of the back. Also, cysts, tumors, and infections may develop in the bones of the spine itself.

In a child who appears to be ill, rapidly developing lower back pain may be a sign of MENINGITIS, especially when there is also fever and vomiting. Not infrequently, neck stiffness and pain will also be present. Immediate medical attention is *mandatory* if meningitis is suspected.

Professional help is necessary when a child complains of back pain from a fall in which the force has been considerable or there is evidence of injury from a blunt object. In such instances the child should be moved *only* by experienced emergency personnel, since possible neurologic damage may be aggravated if a fracture or joint-instability problem already exists.

Back pain may be an early symptom of SPINAL CURVATURE. Scoliosis is a curvature of the spine that may develop during growth spurts. Frequently the young teenagers with this difficulty must wear an orthopedic brace—just at a time when concerns with body image and physical prowess may be at their highest. A lot of parental support and reassurance are required during the period of treatment, which may take several years.

See also: INFLUENZA.

Bacterial infections

Invasion of the organs or tissues of the body by one or more types of pathogenic (disease-causing) bacteria.

Bacteria are single-celled microorganisms so small that over a million can exist on the head of a pin. They are classified in three ways: First, their general shape: coccus (round), bacillus (rodlike), and spirillum (spiral); second, whether or not they retain a Gram stain (a special laboratory dye), a classification method that helps indicate which of various antibiotics are appropriate to treat the specific bacteria; and third, whether the microorganism is aerobic (requires oxygen in order to live) or anaerobic (able to survive without oxygen).

Bacteria exist naturally in soil, in fresh water, and in the sea. They live in the mouth, in the digestive tract, and on the skin—usually without causing any problem. But sometimes they get misplaced and cause trouble. For example, some types of bacteria, harmless in the intestines, can cause considerable irritation in a girl's vagina if careless wiping sweeps the bacteria to the area.

In a suitable environment, such as an open wound, a small number of bacteria can multiply into several million within a relatively short time. The microorganisms generally reproduce by splitting into two identical cells. If you start with one million, you may have two, then three, then four million and more. Some of them are able to form a thick wall around themselves, becoming a cyst or spore that is resistant to heat, drying, or the effects of chemicals intended to kill them.

Most bacterial infections can be treated successfully with one or more of the antibiotic drugs. An antibiotic is a chemical substance produced by certain species of bacteria, molds, or other microorganisms. When it comes in contact with other species of germs, it can kill them or inhibit their growth and multiplication. Antibiotics are among the very few drugs that can cure a disease by removing its cause. Penicillin was one of the first of the modern antibiotics to be discovered, and it is still considered to be one of the most useful in treating a wide range of infections. Today, however, physicians have many different antibiotics to choose from in the treatment of specific bacterial infections.

Not all antibiotics act in the same way, nor are they equally effective against a specific bacterial infection. The one that is prescribed by the child's physician depends on the nature and severity of the infection, whether the child is especially sensitive to the drug (for example, some people are extremely sensitive or allergic to penicillin and may experience ANAPHYLACTIC SHOCK if it is given), and whether the bacteria may have become resistant to a particular antibiotic.

It is very important to see that the child completes the full course of antibiotic therapy exactly as the physician directs. That is, if the doctor says the child should take the drug for ten days, it should not be stopped two or three days after the first dose just because the child seems to look and feel better. Taking too little of the drug or failing to take it at the proper intervals can allow the infection to progress and may also cause an immune effect in the bacteria, so that the antibiotic won't work. This occurs because natural selection allows the stronger microorganisms to predominate so that treatment-resistant strains emerge.

It is also important that the child not be given more of the drug than is prescribed and that doses not be given more frequently than instructed. Either of these overloads may result in annoying or even potentially dangerous side effects. If nothing else, it's costly and ineffective. If treatment is to be effective, the physician's instructions must be followed to the letter. Otherwise recovery time may be greatly prolonged or complications may develop.

Compare VIRAL INFECTIONS.

Bad breath

See BREATH ODOR.

Balding

See HAIR, LOSS AND THINNING.

Bedwetting

When the young child has not even reached the stage of fairly constant daytime control, enuresis (the medical term for bedwetting) is to be expected. Many normal, healthy children continue to wet the bed at night long after they have achieved good daytime control. A parent need have little concern unless the nighttime bedwetting persists much beyond the age of five years—although even then an occasional mishap should probably be overlooked.

Bedwetting seems to be more common among boys. Possibly this reflects a high degree of physical and emotional activity that, in turn, induces such deep sleep that the sphincter muscle that controls the bladder loosens and urine flows.

A hidden urinary tract infection can cause enuresis, and this may be especially true for girls. Although such infections—as well as other medical conditions (an enlarged bladder or kidney; a seizure disorder; certain hormonal imbalances; diabetes)—can cause bedwetting, the parent should be relieved to know that most cases stem from less serious problems. A medical evaluation is suggested so that treatable causes can be taken care of.

Helping children gain nighttime control involves some retraining. Often all that's needed is restricting fluid intake after dinner—limiting children to no more than a few ounces of water—and awakening them to get up and urinate just before parents go to bed.

The old gold-star method may be helpful. Parents and the child should collaborate in keeping a chart that leads to some suitable reward system as progress occurs.

Older children may benefit from having an alarm set to go off just before the time they have generally been found to wet the bed. A degree of responsibility and self-sufficiency can be fostered if these children are provided with dry bed clothing and pajamas and told that they should not disturb their parents during the night.

Some electronic devices are available commercially. One alarm sounds whenever the bed is wet. After a period of several weeks the child is conditioned to respond to bladder fullness before the alarm goes off. Another device hooks directly to the child's pajamas. Its alarm is a buzzer that rests on the child's pillow and awakens only him or her, not the entire household.

Certain methods of bladder training may be suggested by the child's doctor. Parents may be asked to help teach the child during waking hours to retain urine for as long as possible and then record the volume of urine passed. Another alternative is medication, although this is generally not done if the child is under the age of six years and parents must ensure that dose and timing instructions are followed to the letter. Hypnosis is also proving to be an effective method of helping achieve control.

Emotional difficulties must, of course, be considered. The pendulum has swung away from its old direction—that is, the belief that bedwetting is always a symptom of severe psychological disturbance. But stress, anxiety, fear of parental rejection, envy of a younger sibling's bedwetting "privileges," and other factors can play a definite role in children's continuing bedwetting—or regressing to that behavior once they've outgrown it.

For almost all children, nighttime wetting is an embarrassing and demeaning affair. Parents who become so frustrated that they punish, tease, or reprimand only compound the problem. Supportive reassurance works far better than punishment, and parents who take an active part in applying retraining techniques can encourage cooperation on the child's part.

If the situation is not alleviated by some of the techniques mentioned here, professional psychological evaluation is in order. This is especially so when other signs of immaturity such as temper tantrums or late thumb sucking are present. Sometimes hypnosis is effective, but any such treatment should be undertaken only by qualified professionals after a medical evaluation has eliminated the possibility of some organic defect or infectious disease.

Bee stings

See STINGS.

Behavior changes in teenagers

An alteration in the teenager's conduct that is unusual and prolonged enough to bring attention to the fact that there has been a change.

It is a basic characteristic of human beings to have variations in mood and behavior. Everyone has good days and bad days. The reasons for these changes are frequently multiple, but even singly they may be very complex. If we don't feel well physically, if the weather is bad, or if our plans go awry, we may react negatively to those around us. In the same way, when everything goes well, we tend to react positively.

What emerges even with the changes, however, is a pattern of behavior that is fairly consistent and readily observed by others. A child's emerging personality pattern is discernible to parents. Moods can be sensed, and some of the child's reactions are often predictable. It is normal for adolescence to be accompanied by wide mood swings that make it more difficult for parents to monitor the flow of feelings. But alert parents can usually judge how life is going for their child. Being a good observer is a crucial part of parenting. Development of a sense that tells you how your child reacts to stress, for example, will help parents provide support when it's needed. Similarly, parents can develop sensitivity to whether bringing the subject up for discussion may be perceived as invasive and when the child is silently asking the parents to help by sympathetically listening and talking.

Gradual behavior changes toward more social responsibility indicate the child is maturing. For instance, the teenager who has been driving too fast begins to slow down—an indication of accepting adult-level responsibility.

If, on the other hand, parents note accumulating negativity in their adolescent's behavior, it's a sign that the child may be having difficulty handling something stressful. Irritability and fatigability are important signals parents should be aware of. When causes are not obvious or if the unhappiness is persistent, close attention must be paid. It's important for parents to remember that their own negative reactions to a child's negative behavior will only aggravate the situation. Try to develop a tone of support. If your efforts don't succeed, seek the advice of the child's physician.

Very abrupt changes in an adolescent's behavior, whether negative or seemingly positive, require special consideration. A teenager who has been previously withdrawn and acting depressed may become relaxed, even jovial, when he or she reaches a decision to attempt suicide. Deceptively, a teenager's mood may lighten tremendously after deciding to run away from home. These quick changes in mood occur when a person who has been wrestling with a problem for a long time suddenly sees a solution, no matter how dramatic, or even life threatening, that solution may be.

Gradual positive changes are healthy. Negative changes should cause concern. Sudden and unexplained behavior changes, either positive or negative, should be scrutinized carefully.

Birth injuries

Any injury that occurs just before or during the time of an infant's delivery. Some studies suggest that these kinds of injuries may happen in as many as 7 out of every 1,000 births. Most of them occur even with the most expert obstetrical care and are considered unavoidable.

Most babies emerge headfirst. Not uncommonly, especially if the infant is large, the collarbone or clavicle may be fractured. Newborns with fractured collarbones tend not to use the arm on the affected side, or they may cry when the arm is moved. Sometimes swelling and a bluish discoloration will be noticed in the skin that lies over the collarbone area. This injury is not a serious one; the fracture usually heals within two or three weeks. You can offer the infant relief by pinning the sleeve of his or her undershirt across the chest; this helps immobilize the shoulder, which lessens the discomfort.

Fractures of other bones may occur which are noticed shortly after birth. Treatment is undertaken by the medical team attending the birth.

Sometimes when a considerable amount of traction has been required to get the baby out in a hurry, nerves coming from the spinal cord or in an extremity may be injured, in which case parents may notice that the baby will not use the affected limb normally. Recovery of nerve function will depend on whether the nerves were torn or just stretched.

By far the most common site of injury is the head. The infant's head sustains a considerable amount of pressure as the mother's uterine contractions push the baby through the cervix and down the birth canal. The scalp may be swollen and discolored in places, and the skull may appear elongated or pointy. This condition is called molding, and it usually clears up within a few weeks. However, on rare occasions the head injury may be severe enough to cause a skull fracture or bleeding into the brain. Should this happen the baby will quickly develop symptoms that will alert the nurses and doctors to start therapy. The nature of that therapy will depend on the degree of involvement, but modern techniques of treating tiny infants have substantially lowered the rates of death or serious impairment.

Rather frequently a localized area of bleeding occurs on a baby's skull; it looks like a large bump or goose egg. The blood that causes these bumps is usually absorbed by the baby's body in two to three weeks. On occasion the lump may last longer. No treatment is required, and parents need not be concerned.

Sometimes a small, bright red area of bleeding shows in the white of a newborn baby's eyes because of pressures which occur on the head during normal birth processes. This, too, should cause no parental concern. It clears up by itself.

Similarly, parents need not worry about the scrapes, scratches, or under-the-skin lumps that may occur when forceps have been used to assist in delivery. They, too, clear up in a short time.

Birthmarks

Approximately 40 percent of infants are born with one type or another of localized, discolored areas on the skin. Generally known as birthmarks, they occur because early in the baby's intrauterine development, certain elements in the blood-vessel system fail to unite properly. Usually these lesions are not associated with any other abnormality.

The most common types of birthmarks are called HEMANGIOMAS. They may range from faint reddened areas on the skin to larger denser masses which show some elevation above the skin surface. Therapy, if any is needed, will depend on the type of hemangioma present.

Nevus pigmentosus (a mole) is a brown-colored mark that may be present at birth or may develop later in childhood. Most authorities now believe that those moles present at birth should be removed sometime before young adulthood. Any mole that blisters, bleeds, darkens, or changes in any way should be examined by a physician to make sure no malignant growth is involved.

Bites

See ANIMAL BITES, HUMAN BITES, INSECT BITES, SNAKEBITES, SPIDER BITES, TICK BITES.
Compare STINGS.

Bleeding problem

See BLOOD IN THE STOOLS, BLOOD IN THE URINE, BLOOD IN THE VOMITUS, BRUISE, HEMOPHILIA.

Blisters

A raised, watery sac on the skin or the lining of the mouth. Blisters are a reaction of the uppermost layers of the skin either to an injury from pressure or heat or to a bacterial or viral infection.

Heat injuries, including sunburn and burns and scalds, may cause extensive blistering of the skin. The affected areas should be cleansed with an antibacterial soap several times a day; when the injuries are extensive, they should be treated by a physician. Make no attempt to rupture the blister; in time the fluid will be released as the underlying skin heals. Special antibiotic creams may be necessary, and care to prevent infection is imperative. Pressure blisters, usually on the hands and feet, require no special care except cleansing and placing a soft dressing over the skin to prevent further injury. A nonstick pad put directly in contact with the blister allows for ease of removal.

Cold sores (blisters on the lips) are caused by a particular virus, *herpes simplex.* The blister usually heals in eight to ten days and requires no therapy. Occasionally an impetigo may develop from a cold sore. The original spot will become crusted and not heal, and other sores will begin to develop around the initial one. Consult the child's physician, since an oral antibiotic may be needed.

When children run high fevers—temperatures of up to 105°F (40.5°C)—blisters inside the mouth may indicate viral illnesses such as HERPETIC STOMATITIS or HERPANGINA. Despite their impressive names, neither of these diseases is serious and they usually clear up by themselves in seven to ten days. However, when the child's fever is still high and the illness is in full swing, he or she may suffer considerable pain in the throat and mouth, as well as generalized aching and discomfort. Parents can help by administering plenty of cool liquids, aspirin or acetaminophen, and using a cotton swab to dab a soothing, nonburning preparation such as Gly-Oxide on the blisters.

Newborn infants with a blistering type of diaper rash may be infected with the staphylococcal germ. Prompt medical attention is necessary because of the potential need for antibiotic therapy.

Although rare, there are several congenital (present-at-birth) skin diseases that show blistering as a predominant sign. The physician's diagnosis—and subsequent treatment—are based on the frequency and severity of the skin lesions.

Blindness

In the strict sense of the word, blindness is total loss of vision. In both the practical and legal senses, however, blindness usually includes visual defects that are so severe that certain forms of activity or eventual employment are difficult or impossible.

In some cases there may be some perception of light, but the images formed on the child's retina are hazy and dim. Some types of blindness or partial blindness can be corrected with prompt medical or surgical attention. In other cases early treatment can arrest or slow the progress of defective eyesight that could lead to blindness. Parents should be sure that their children receive thorough eye examinations at whatever interval the pediatrician or family doctor suggests.

Of late there has been considerable attention paid to the disease called retinitis pigmentosa, which is thought to be hereditary and which eventually leads to blindness. In children who are affected, opthalmoscopic examination by an eye doctor will generally show abnormalities by the time the child is ten years old. Poor night vision may be evident much earlier, so parents who notice that their children have unusual difficulty seeing at night will want to have the children's eyes examined at once.

Causes of blindness include congenital (present-at-birth) defects of the eye, the optic nerve, or the visual center of the brain; wounds and other injuries; increased pressure within the skull; degeneration or detachment of the retina; eye or brain tumors; severe diabetes; meningitis (an inflammation of the membranes covering the brain); or complications stemming from chronic inflammation of the eye.

Blood in the stools

Sometimes called rectal bleeding, blood in the stools generally indicates that either an irritation or a structural abnormality exists somewhere along the digestive tract. Unlike ANAL FISSURES, rectal bleeding requires a thorough medical evaluation. Some confusion may arise when children have consumed beets, certain fruits, artificially colored drinks, or other foods that will cause a red or purple discoloration in a child's bowel movement. If there is a clear history of this kind of food intake, and the situation does not recur until the next purplish-red meal, parents need not be alarmed. But if there is any doubt, a simple chemical test done in a doctor's office can confirm the nature of the liquid or solid discoloration.

Note the amount, the frequency and the color of the bleeding so that an accurate report can be made to the doctor. Blood coming from high in the digestive tract—that is, from the mouth, throat, esophagus, or stomach—will have a black, thick, sticky appearance: the so-called tarry stool. This dark discoloration is caused by stomach acid and other processes that play a role in digestion. Blood swallowed from a nosebleed may also produce tarry stools.

Blood-streaked mucus may show up in the bowel movements of children—especially young infants—who have acute GASTROENTERITIS, a common viral illness that inflames the stomach and intestines. In these instances there is not a great deal of blood and the bleeding subsides when the child stops vomiting and suffering diarrhea.

Bloody diarrhea may occur with certain bacterial infections of the intestines such as salmonella or shigella. Usually the child will also have a fever over 102°F. Most commonly, these disorders clear up by themselves, although occasionally antibiotic therapy may be necessary. Bloody diarrhea also frequently accompanies inflammatory intestinal diseases such as REGIONAL ENTERITIS and COLITIS. In severe cases abdominal cramping, weight loss, and fatigability from anemia are prominent features.

Bright red blood mixed with a bowel movement can occur from a MECKEL'S DIVERTICULUM or, more often, as the result of an intestinal polyp (a small growth). These little growths are most often found in the lower section of the intestinal tract and a physician will use an instrument called a sigmoidoscope to inspect them and sometimes take a biopsy specimen. Children's polyps are very rarely malignant, and the doctor may choose not even to remove them. However, especially if they are large, they may cause a rather copious amount of bright red rectal bleeding, which may be alarming to the parent and to the child. However disconcerting the situation, it is rarely a dangerous one. Only when there is a family history of multiple polyps, and the child shows the same tendency, need any extensive surgery be undertaken.

Occasionally bleeding from the intestinal tract may be so slow that no blood is noticed in the child's stools. The diagnosis will usually be made while a physician is searching for the cause of anemia. INTUSSUSCEPTION may cause rectal bleeding that shows up as a thick, stringy bowel movement called currant jelly stool.

As noted, blood in the stool may occur in a number of illnesses that are not serious, or the "blood" may be nothing more than coloring from some food or drink. But, on occasion, there may be blood loss that warrants specific therapy, or an illness or structural abnormality that needs prompt medical attention. So when parents first suspect rectal bleeding, they should certainly consult with a doctor.

Blood in the urine

Technically known as hematuria, blood in the urine is not common in children. If the child's urine appears reddish or tea colored, parents should first carefully review what the youngster had to eat or drink in the previous twelve to twenty-four hours. For example, beets or artificial food colorings may cause an unusual color in the urine. However, if you are at all uncertain, check with a doctor. A simple chemical test done in the doctor's office will clarify whether blood is actually present.

Blood in the urine, which generally also contains pus cells the doctor can note by microscope, may occur in urinary tract infections. Parents may begin to suspect this condition if the child makes frequent trips to the bathroom and complains of discomfort on urination. The treatment generally consists of oral antibiotics.

Children with nephritis (kidney inflammation) tend to pass a dark red or brown urine. In one form of this disease, acute glomerulonephritis, infrequent urination may be a symptom and the child will show swelling of body parts, especially the eyelids and, in males, the scrotum. Once the diagnosis is made, treatment most likely includes the restriction of fluids. Generally speaking, the kidneys heal in a period of several weeks and the child suffers no long-term harm.

Injuries may also cause bloody urine, as can happen if there is a tear in kidney tissue caused by a direct blow to either of the kidney areas. So-called ammonia burns—inflamed areas at the tip of the penis—may cause small amounts of bleeding that seem to be coming with urination. Frequent application of a protective cream allows these so-called burns to heal, and no further treatment is needed. An inflammation of tissues around the vaginal opening may be responsible for blood that appears to accompany the flow of urine in girls. In both boys and girls, direct injury to the genitals may cause bright red bleeding. A medical examination is a must to ensure that no serious tears are present.

On occasion, small amounts of blood in the urine may not be noticed at all, but they may be detected when tests are done as part of a routine physical examination. When this occurs, other signs and symptoms of illness, as well as family history, will be used by the physician to reach a diagnosis.

Since there are any number of conditions that may be associated with blood in the urine, parents should not delay seeking medical advice if their children show any evidence of such bleeding.

Blood in the vomitus

The appearance of small amounts of bright red blood in the fluids a child vomits frequently arises from an irritation at the back of the nose or throat. On occasion, prolonged or particularly forceful retching tears the small blood vessels in the esophagus (the swallowing channel), which produces tiny patches of blood in the child's vomitus.

Before the parent becomes unduly concerned, it's a good idea to review what the child has eaten or drunk over the previous several hours. Red dyes used in food and drink colorings, as well as certain foods themselves, may be the real source of what appears to be blood. If there's any doubt, a simple chemical test done in a doctor's office or an emergency room will settle the question.

Parents may also want to carefully monitor their children when they take seemingly harmless drugs such as aspirin. Aspirin can irritate the stomach and cause bleeding that may be vomited.

When a child suffers a nosebleed, fairly large amounts of blood may be swallowed. If the blood remains in the stomach for even a short period of time, it may be regurgitated as a dark-colored coffee grounds material. The coffee grounds consistency and a dark brown to black color may also characterize blood vomited when the child has a peptic ulcer or some other problem involving the esophagus or stomach. If more than a tablespoon of such vomitus appears, urgent medical evaluation is necessary. Coffee ground vomitus is a classic sign of cancer of the stomach, although parents should be reassured that children are very rarely afflicted with that disorder.

If there is internal bleeding that is brisk, the vomitus is bright red. Here, too, parents should seek immediate medical attention.

Certain caustic poisons, if eaten or drunk, cause severe burning of the upper intestinal tract, resulting in the vomiting of blood. If there is any reason to suspect the child has ingested such a substance, call for immediate emergency assistance and also contact the nearest Poison Control Center for advice about first-aid procedures. Parents should keep this number beside the telephone at all times. You can get the number from the appendix in this book (see p. 317).

Blood poisoning

See SEPTICEMIA.

Blood pressure

Blood pressure tends to vary according to a person's body position, level of activity, and other factors, but a school-age child's systolic and diastolic (top and bottom) blood pressure measurements should probably never exceed 100/80 or 110/80.

Up until and including about the age of four, an average reading is 85/60. Then, for a while, the top figure increases approximately 5 points with every two years of age added.

age 6	90/60
age 8	95/62
age 10	100/65

The increase then slows until the adolescent is about sixteen.

age 12	108/67
age 14	112/70
age 16	118/75

Bloodshot eyes

See EYE REDNESS.

Blood sugar, low

See HYPOGLYCEMIA.

Bloody nose

See NOSEBLEED.

Blueness of the skin

See CYANOSIS.

Blurred vision

A defect in which the child sees an unfocused blur when an image is focused on the retina. This partial or total blurring can result from eye injuries, eye infections, certain diseases or structural defects of the eye or optic nerve, and may also occur as a side effect from prescription or over-the-counter drugs. Because it is essential that the underlying cause be determined and, if possible, treated or corrected, parents should not attempt to treat such a condition. If the child complains of blurred vision or younger, nonverbal youngsters seem to have trouble focusing on objects, they should immediately be taken to a physician or eye specialist who can determine what is wrong.

See also: FARSIGHTEDNESS, NEARSIGHTEDNESS.

Body rocking

See ROCKING.

Body temperature

The heat of the human body, measured in degrees Fahrenheit (°F) or degrees Celsius or Centigrade (°C). The average body temperature, taken by mouth with a clinical thermometer, is 98.6°F (37°C). However, this figure may vary slightly from one individual to another, or at different times during the day, or when extreme activity or noticeable change in air temperature causes variations that can be considered normal.

This variation in children's body temperature is particularly noticeable in newborn babies, especially if they are premature or sick. Newborns can be affected not only by the temperature of the air but also by humidity, air flow, and the temperature of surfaces they're in contact with—for example, bedclothing or a mattress.

Until a child is old enough to be relied upon to hold a thermometer under his or her tongue, a youngster's temperature should be taken rectally or under the armpit. The parent should keep in mind, however, that a rectal temperature can be expected to read about 1°F higher than one taken orally; an axillary (under-the-armpit) temperature may read about 1°F or 2°F lower than an oral temperature.

Parents whose children customarily show slight variations in body temperatures without showing any signs of illness need not be unduly alarmed. They may wish to keep track of these variations and perhaps tie them to certain environmental or activity factors before consulting their physician about whether the child should be professionally examined.

See also: FEVER, HYPOTHERMIA.

Boils

A pus-filled inflammation, called a furuncle, of an infected hair follicle or sebaceous (oil-secreting) gland.

Bacteria may use small breaks in the skin's surface to cause many kinds of skin disorders. When they burrow through to hair roots or sebaceous glands, they may cause a walled-off area of infection that becomes red, tender, and filled with pus: a boil.

The most common sites for boils are on the face, the back of the neck, under the arms, and the lower part of the back. Cleanliness, daily changing of clothes, and the use of an antibacterial soap may reduce the likelihood of children getting boils, although some youngsters seem unusually prone to them, especially as they reach puberty and the sebaceous glands are more active.

Boils sometimes disappear spontaneously after three or four days. They should *never* be picked at, squeezed, or pierced at home by the parent or the child because this may cause the bacteria, frequently staphylococcal germs, to spread to other places, including the bloodstream, which could lead to a form of blood poisoning called SEPTICEMIA. Warm compresses may help bring the boil to a head and also relieve the pain.

If a boil persists or increases in size, it is best to have a physician pierce it to release the pus before a dressing is applied. In some cases antibiotic therapy may be prescribed.

Compare CARBUNCLE.

Botulism

A potentially fatal form of food poisoning caused by a toxin produced when *Clostridium botulinum* grows in improperly preserved foods. Concern has arisen that infants may contract botulism and its serious consequences from honey used as food or formula sweetner. Recent evidence suggests that commercial corn syrups may also contain the toxin in amounts harmful to babies. It is recommended that honey or syrup sweetner not be given to infants under 12 months old.

See also: FOOD POISONING.

Bowel movement

It is important for parents to understand their child's usual bowel movement pattern so they can notice any change that may signal the need to consult a physician.

The bowel movements of a newborn baby may be green and sticky for the first few days. This is caused by meconium (a substance created in the baby's intestinal tract while the infant is in the uterus). Transitional stools—a mixture of green and yellow—will then follow.

During the first few months of life, babies tend to have as many as five or six yellow, "seedy," watery bowel movements a day. This pattern will be especially true for breast-fed infants—although it is also seen in babies taking formulas—and it simply means that the young baby is efficiently using all the milk being taken in, so that there is little left but water to excrete.

On the other hand, infants may reabsorb all the water and fluids from their diet; when this happens, the baby may go for a day or two without dirtying a diaper. Sometimes an infant may shift between these two patterns. However, if three days go by without a bowel movement, stimulating the rectum with a lubricated thermometer or a glycerin suppository may be required to cause a movement. If this does not work, do *not* give the infant a laxative of any sort. Consult the baby's doctor at once. Although the condition is rare, sometimes the last portion of a very young baby's intestinal tract does not move correctly and the infant cannot evacuate unless surgically treated.

As the infant grows and begins eating solid food, a more definite bowel movement pattern is established. Usually one to three yellow to brown movements will be passed each day. The stools will be pasty to firm, and the odor and color will depend on what the child has eaten.

When toilet training is achieved, and especially by the time a child starts school, the usual pattern is that of one or two soft but well-formed bowel movements a day. Parents should remember, however, that variations may occur when there are diet changes—for example, high intake of fluids or eating too much or too little fiber.

Parents are frequently concerned when babies and youngsters show signs of discomfort as they have a bowel movement. Bright red faces, grunting noises, and occasional crying are common signs. If the stool appears normal once it is passed, parents need not be concerned. This straining process is nature's way of helping the baby increase the abdominal pressure that is necessary to pass a normal bowel movement. When the stool appears hard and pelletlike, parents can give the child one of the commercially available stool softeners, in either milk or water, to help loosen the consistency of the movement. This quantity can be increased to two tablespoonfuls a day if the problem persists. When the child's stools are soft and easily passed, taper off the softener, or consult a doctor for advice about whether to continue, stop, or switch to some other method if necessary.

Once parents understand the child's usual pattern(s), they can be more accurate in noticing changes. DIARRHEA could signal the presence of an acute infection. Bloody diarrhea, especially when abdominal pain is present, might indicate REGIONAL ENTERITIS or COLITIS. CONSTIPATION, especially when it is chronic, should generally be evaluated by a doctor before any therapy is started. Laxatives should *never* be given to the child. In addition to irritating the intestinal tract, they may cause a dependency called the laxative habit, which leads to the use of stronger and stronger medications. In some cases, such as appendicitis, the use of laxatives can cause extreme harm.

BLOOD IN THE STOOLS, ABDOMINAL BLOATING, VOMITING, and black, tarry movements are some signs that indicate the presence of a significant disease; the child needs to be examined by a physician. Very light colored or white stools may be found in HEPATITIS. Green, slimy bowel movements with mucus in them may indicate swallowed drainage from some upper respiratory disorder, or possibly some disease affecting the intestinal tract. Foul-smelling, fatty stools that float on the toilet water may be found in CYSTIC FIBROSIS and in a MALABSORPTION SYNDROME. Children who have been placed on a liquid diet may, after two or three days, expel green, watery movements called starvation stools.

When parents cannot readily tie children's changed bowel movement patterns to diet, fluid intake, or minor viral infections, they should consult a physician.

Bowlegs

A condition in which the knees bow outward, appearing too widely separated, and cannot be closed when the feet are together. Sometimes there is a family history of bowlegs. Very rarely does the condition restrict or limit movement.

Bowlegs are extremely common in infants and toddlers. The defect usually corrects itself within about one year after the child begins to walk. The child's doctor will generally become concerned only if the condition is unusually severe or if it occurs out of its normal sequence in the growth pattern. Shoes wedges are generally not prescribed because they accomplish little if anything and, in fact, may make the child's feet uncomfortable.

Certain congenital (present-at-birth) diseases of bone formation as well as rickets acquired later in childhood may cause an unusual degree of bowing. On very rare occasions a disorder known as Blount's disease causes bowlegs. The diagnosis is made by X ray, and the defect may require bracing or even surgery for correction.

Brain infection

See ENCEPHALITIS, MENINGITIS.

Breast enlargement, male

See GYNECOMASTIA.

Breasts

Newborn infants often show puffed-out breasts. This condition is caused by the temporary hormonal influences from the mother's blood. Within a few weeks the engorgement disappears on its own. No treatment is needed, and parents can simply relax and reassure themselves that there is nothing wrong with the baby.

Female breasts begin to develop at puberty, although they may occur earlier and should cause no concern unless other secondary sexual characteristics also make an early appearance, in which case medical attention should be sought. Some teenage girls are worried by one of two concerns: their breasts seem to be either too small or too large. Occasionally, if a girl is unduly preoccupied by what she perceives as underdevelopment or overdevelopment, she may wish to discuss the matter with a physician or psychologist. More often than not, some reassurance from her mother and her own gradual learning that breasts are by no means the sole key to attractiveness enable the female adolescent to overcome her shyness and concern.

Especially during adolescence, both girls and boys may complain of a lump under one or both of the nipples. It occurs because tissue in that location is sensitive to *normal* amounts of the hormone estrogen. The area may be tender if touched or struck, but the condition is not harmful and generally disappears in a period of weeks. Only if the area gradually enlarges need medical evaluation be sought, and then regularly scheduled checkups might be recommended.

Bleeding from the nipple is almost always due to a benign (harmless) condition that generally is corrected by surgery. (Discharge from the nipple can also occur when cysts are present, but the secretions are not bloodstained.)

Fibroadenoma is a common disease of the breast. It usually occurs during the period from puberty to thirty years of age. In young girls the tumors are firm and rubbery, easily moved about within the breast tissue and slipping away from the physician's examining fingers. They rarely grow to a large size, and they never develop into cancer. Neither does their occurrence increase the chances of cancer developing at a later time. The treatment is the same as for any distinct lump in the breast: it is removed surgically and examined very carefully to make absolutely sure there is no cancer involved. When the lump is removed, there is usually no disfiguration whatsoever, the scar is completely unnoticeable, and recurrences are rare.

Mastitis is the name given to an infection and inflammation of the breasts. It is most likely to occur during breast-feeding, when germs may enter through cracks babies may make when they suck on the nipples, but the disorder can occur at any age. The microorganisms that cause the infection are *Staphylococci*, the same type of germ that causes common skin infections such as BOILS. Antibiotics can clear up the infection within a relatively short time, especially if given early. If treatment is delayed, an abscess may form, which leads to a swelling under a reddened area of skin. If this happens, a small incision may have to be made in the breast so the fluid can be drained.

Compare GYNECOMASTIA.

Breath holding

A form of behavior in which an infant or young child—usually in the toddler stage—consciously holds his or her breath. This usually occurs as a response to frustration, an expression of anger, or a kind of testing of newfound abilities much as temper tantrums are.

The color of the youngster's face goes from red to purple

to blue. The event may proceed to a point where the child does, in fact, stop breathing for a moment or two, usually not longer than one minute, at which time there may be a loss of consciousness. However, should this occur, nature's protective mechanism comes into play and the child starts breathing again spontaneously—just as we breathe when we are asleep because parts of our brain and respiratory system work without our conscious control.

If the episode is a long one, twitching movements or even CONVULSIONS are possible. However frightening—even terrifying—the event may be for the parent, there are no harmful or long-term effects from a breath-holding spell.

An old recommendation to parents was that they ignore such outbursts and perhaps even leave the room. This seems unwise. Children in this state ought to be observed. If the color changes progress to white or ashen and the child is not breathing, mouth-to-mouth resuscitation should be started. In more extreme cases, if the heartbeat or pulse are absent, full cardiopulmonary resuscitation should be undertaken. As pointed out elsewhere, one should not begin cardiac massage unless the heart has stopped. So a good rule for parents to follow is: simply observe the child to make sure nothing untoward is happening; otherwise, just let the episode continue through its stages, giving it no special attention and never intervening to try to stop it by shaking or holding the child.

Children should not be allowed to acquire the habit of breath holding because they sense it is an effective emotional tool useful to defy parental control. At the earliest opportunity, discuss the problem with the child's doctor. Perhaps special tests such as an electroencephalogram may be warranted to make sure there is no neurological or other medical component present. If parents can determine what kinds of events seem to kick off such behavior, perhaps they can be avoided. However, they should not give children their own way just to avoid frustration that culminates in a breath-holding spell. A physician's or psychologist's advice may be helpful to parents confronted by the dilemma of what to do and what not to do. Fortunately, in most instances toddlers outgrow this behavior when they learn that there are more socially acceptable ways to express their frustration.

Breathing difficulties

When children experience difficulties with breathing, it is often associated with a stuffy nose—nasal congestion from the common cold.

However, at times children may make a whistling type of sound when they breathe. This wheezing usually means that the airways to the lungs are obstructed with thick secretions or the presence of some foreign object. Medical evaluation is clearly needed.

Among the many possible causes of breathing difficulties in children are ASTHMA, CROUP, and PNEUMONIA. Accidental poisoning or an overdose of aspirin are others. Since parents lacking medical training are in no position to make an accurate diagnosis and start the most appropriate treatment, children who are having breathing difficulties—without a stuffy nose—should be taken to a doctor immediately.

Young infants may turn blue or start choking when they experience a breathing difficulty. On occasion this may signal underlying medical problems that could lead to SUDDEN INFANT DEATH SYNDROME. If a qualified physician determines that such abnormalities are present, parents may wish to install a special alarm system that will allow them to monitor their child's breathing and alert them to any sudden difficulty.

Breath odor

Medically known as halitosis, breath odor in children can usually be traced to poor dental hygiene or tooth decay. Children should be taught to brush and floss so that a buildup of plaque doesn't occur. Dental plaque houses bacteria that can cause decay, further adding to bad breath.

Other unpleasant mouth odors can occur with disease. For example, an acute or chronic infection of the tonsils or back part of the child's nose may result in bad breath. Foreign bodies previously placed in the nose by the child may cause such an infection and be responsible for an infected-looking drainage as well as the bad breath. DIABETES MELLITUS and other disturbances in metabolism can cause the breath to have the odor of acetone, which smells rather like an open bottle of fingernail-polish remover. On rare occasions breath may smell like ammonia or urine if a child's kidneys are not functioning properly; but this is a late sign and by that time so many other symptoms will have appeared that the child will undoubtedly be in treatment, so this type of bad breath may never develop.

Breathing rate

As an exchange of oxygen and carbon dioxide takes place in the lungs, adults breathe in and out approximately sixteen times each minute.

The breathing rate of children is typically higher than that of adults. This rate will vary, depending on the child's physical activity, state of wakefulness or sleepiness, comfort or discomfort, and various emotional factors. As a general guide for parents who may be interested, children's rates tend to follow these ranges:

Age	Expected range (breaths per minute)
Newborns	30–40
Infants	20–100
1 year–adulthood	20

Parents should note that these figures are for expected *ranges;* the actual rate may vary from minute to minute. If your child's breathing rate is *consistently* over 40 per minute, there may be some heart or lung problem, and medical consultation is recommended.

See also: BREATHING DIFFICULTIES, PNEUMONIA.
Compare HEART RATE.

Brittle nails

See NAILS.

Bronchiolitis

An acute inflammation of the bronchioles (the very tiny breathing tubes in the lungs) that causes a cough and wheezing. In most cases the disease is caused by a virus, and it is most common during the winter and early spring months.

Although the disorder is seen in youngsters as old as two, it usually affects babies under the age of eighteen months, commonly around the age of six months.

The first symptoms are usually a runny nose, a low-grade fever, and other signs of an upper respiratory infection. The cough that develops becomes progressively worse, and the child begins to wheeze. The breathing rate may increase from a normal average of 30 times per minute up to as high as 80.

A physician's evaluation is necessary because breathing distress may progress to the point at which the affected baby may turn blue. Babies with bronchiolitis are often hospitalized so they can be properly oxygenated. An oxygen tent with mist will allow moisture to loosen mucous secretions and make the breathing effort easier. Hospitalization also permits professional suctioning of this mucus, as some babies may tend to choke on their own secretions.

Since bronchiolitis is a viral illness, not a bacterial one, antibiotics are of no value unless bacterial PNEUMONIA complicates the situation. Within a few days the wheezing lessens, and by a week to ten days the baby is well. After recovery babies may cough for several days, but the coughing is not associated with respiratory distress.

It used to be thought that bronchiolitis would not recur in a child who has once had it. However, it now seems that babies who have had bronchiolitis do show an increased tendency to wheeze when they are stricken with other viruses that cause upper-respiratory ailments. But other than that, the disease seems to leave no long-term ill effects.

Bronchitis

Inflammation of the bronchi, the large air passages that lead to the lungs. It can be chronic or acute, but most infants or children suffer from acute bronchitis.

Tiredness, poor nutrition, and exposure to cold, wet, or fog seem to trigger the disease. Young children who live in damp, foggy climates are particularly susceptible. Bronchitis can be caused by infection from a virus, bacteria, or even a fungus. In the tropics a parasitic worm may be the culprit. It can also occur as a complication of some other illness such as whooping cough or measles, or it may be due to an allergy to irritating substances such as smoke (including cigarette smoke), dust, and some gases.

Smoking can greatly increase the risk of acute bronchitis (as well as other diseases that interfere with normal lung function), so older children experimenting with cigarette smoking should be strongly urged not to take that risk. Studies also indicate that children of parents who smoke have a higher incidence of respiratory problems.

Bronchitis strikes suddenly, and the bronchial tubes react the same way as nasal passages do to a cold: they become dry, then "runny," then they gradually return to normal. The child may complain of chest discomfort that seems to be located behind the breastbone. A dry, irritating, hacking cough gradually loosens as the passages become more moist. At that time children old enough to spit out what they cough up will generally expectorate a thick, pus-tinged sputum. This is a protective mechanism and explains why most physicians are reluctant to prescribe cough syrups or antihistamines that may suppress the cough reflex.

Occasionally doctors may advise parents to construct "croup tents" over their infant's crib so that a cold-steam humidifier can moisten the air. In most cases parents will be advised merely to make sure the child gets plenty of fluids, rest, and perhaps moderate doses of aspirin to relieve fever—which, if present, is generally not too high. Antibiotics are not indicated unless the illness is caused by or accompanied by bacterial infection.

In most instances acute bronchitis is mild and does not last more than a few days. However, children who suffer repeated attacks should receive a careful medical evaluation.

Bronchopneumonia

See PNEUMONIA.

Bruise

A bruise, medically known as a contusion, is a tissue injury caused by a sudden impact or crushing injury. The skin remains unbroken, but discoloration results from the rupturing of tiny blood vessels.

Pain and swelling commonly follow a severe bruise. Massive contusions, such as may result from a blow to the head or a fractured skull, require immediate medical attention! For minor bruises, parents can administer first aid by intermittently applying cold, wet compresses; an ice bag; or fresh-water ice. Salt-water ice should be avoided because the temperature of the slush will be low enough to cause further tissue damage. The child should rest the injured part so that blood flow will not be increased by activity. After about twenty-four hours a heating pad or hot wet dressings can be used. If the bruise does not improve in two days, or if it continues to increase in size, medical attention is important.

Many parents become concerned about the ease with which their children bruise. Black-and-blue marks on the legs are fairly common as a result of bumps and falls suffered during normal play and physical activity. However, if the child goes to bed with no apparent marks and gets up with bruises, especially on the back or chest, a medical difficulty involving spontaneous bleeding may be present. This situation warrants immediate medical attention.

Bulimia

An abnormal increase in the urge to eat; excessive eating. More common in females than males, the condition is thought to be associated with various underlying psychological or sociological causes, which may demand professional help. In typical cases the sufferer lies to others about food intake, secretly gorges on food, and then induces vomiting by sticking a finger down the throat.

The emotional causes of bulimia are not easily resolved, but if the motivation is sufficiently strong and the victim has the understanding of the immediate family or very close friends, the outlook is promising. This condition is frequently associated with a distorted and unrealistic view of the victim's own body image and sense of personal worth.

Compare ANOREXIA NERVOSA.

Burns and scalds

A burn is an injury to body tissue caused by heat, electricity, or chemicals. The severity of a burn depends on how deeply the tissues are affected and what percentage of the total body surface is involved. Scalds are caused when steam or a boiling liquid strikes the skin. The effects are similar to those of any burn, and deeper layers of the tissues may be involved.

Children are very prone to getting burned as they experiment with their own increased mobility, investigate interesting-looking things they may want to touch, or, quite literally, play with fire.

Burns are traditionally classified according to the degree of tissue damage. First-degree burns involve only the epidermis (the outer layer of skin), and are limited to reddening. Second-degree burns involve both the epidermis and the dermis (the inner layer of skin) and they blister. Third-degree burns involve not only the epidermis and dermis but also the tissues below the skin; the skin itself may be charred black, or it may appear pale white.

Third-degree burns are a medical emergency! All third-degree burns and any burn that affects more than 10 percent of a child's body surface demand immediate hospitalization. SHOULD YOUR CHILD BE BURNED IN THIS WAY, CALL AN AMBULANCE OR TAKE THE CHILD TO A HOSPITAL EMERGENCY ROOM WITHOUT DELAY!

As a good rule, parents should not attempt to home-treat *any* burns except minor ones that cover only a small area and quite clearly are no worse than second degree.

Currently accepted first-aid treatment, for first- and second-degree burns, is to apply very cold wet compresses of fresh water. The affected area may also be immersed in cool water or placed under running cold water, although the latter may further damage skin if the stream is too fast and forceful. These measures help relieve pain and they may also minimize tissue destruction or the formation of blisters. It is best not to apply any ointment unless the child's physician advises otherwise. Minor burns are also best left open to the air rather than being covered by any bandage or dressing. The old remedies of greasy materials such as butter or lard should never be used. The doctor may, however, recommend application of some water-soluble antiseptic that also has anesthetic (pain-killing) effects.

Again, parents should keep in mind that severe burns or scalds, especially when they involve large areas of a child's body, can be life threatening. Fluid loss, bacterial infection, and many other factors come into play.

C

Cancer

The catch-all word for various types of malignancies that have in common an abnormal, distorted, or uncontrolled growth of body cells. In some instances these cells are confined to a highly localized area, where the tumorous growth can be removed surgically. In many instances metastasis (spreading) takes place; the malignant cells may be carried by the bloodstream or lymphatic system to body areas far from the original or primary site.

Radiation, implantation of a radioactive substance, and chemotherapy (the administration of drugs that attack and destroy cancer cells) are common treatments, although they are frequently used in conjunction with surgery.

Of the many different malignancies, leukemia and bone cancer seem disproportionately common in children.

During childhood years the most prevalent solid tumors are the neuroblastoma, the ganglioneuroma, and Wilms's tumor. The neuroblastoma and the ganglioneuroma (abnormal growths that can arise anywhere in the nervous system) most commonly occur in the adrenal gland, which is located near the kidney. Neuroblastomas usually occur between infancy and six years.

Wilms's tumor, which affects the kidney, usually occurs in children who are between six months and three years of age.

Neither a neuroblastoma nor a Wilms's tumor is marked by classic symptoms that make diagnosis easy. They are generally discovered when a doctor performs a physical examination and discovers an abdominal mass. Surgery, radiation, and chemotherapy are used as treatments. Cure rates are higher for a Wilms's tumor than for a neuroblastoma. However, when a neuroblastoma or ganglioneuroma is neatly encapsulated, surgical removal may carry a higher success rate.

Cancer of the bone—of which pain is the most prominent symptom—includes giant cell sarcoma, fibrosarcoma, osteogenic sarcoma, Ewing's sarcoma, and multiple myeloma. In most instances surgery is the primary treatment. Sometimes children may have to lose a limb, but if there has been no spread, they may survive into healthy old age.

LEUKEMIA, by far the most common cancer in children and by far the one best known to parents, is a disease in which too many underdeveloped white blood cells take over, so that the bone marrow cannot produce enough red blood cells and other elements normally present in the blood.

Young children between three and five are usually the victims although, of course, leukemia can occur at any age, up through adulthood. Parents may notice a child's listlessness, paleness, proneness to infections (often with fever), and unexplained bruising (caused by heavy bleeding of small vessels).

Laboratory examination will show various abnormalities of the blood, usually including a large increase in white blood cells, but the most accurate diagnosis will be made from a specialist's analysis of bone marrow. Newer forms of chemotherapy have improved the rate of remission (a time when the child is mostly free of symptoms), and now about half the children stricken with leukemia survive more than five years after diagnosis.

Supportive therapy or group talk sessions can be helpful to parents of children with leukemia or any form of cancer. When the child is in remission, he or she should be allowed to engage in normal activities as long as a doctor approves.

Candidiasis

See THRUSH, VAGINITIS, YEAST INFECTION.

Canker sores

Painful open small ulcers (sores) that form on the lips or tissues inside the mouth; they may occur alone or in groups. They are not particularly common in children, although when they do appear they tend to recur (as happens with adults).

The cause may be connected to dietary deficiencies, particularly vitamin B_{12} and folic acid; allergies; infectious microorganisms; or emotional stress, although most often no cause can be determined.

Canker sores ordinarily heal by themselves within one or two weeks. It is not a serious condition, although it may temporarily interfere with a child's eating habits. If the child is particularly bothered by the pain and discomfort, a physician may prescribe a painkiller that can be applied directly to the sore.

Carbuncle

A bacterial skin infection that looks like a collection of boils, except that the infection extends over a wide area and affects deeper layers of skin. Carbuncles, too, are most frequently caused by *Staphylococcus* bacteria, but they take much longer to heal than boils do and the infection may cause more damage to underlying tissues.

Because of the seriousness of the infections, carbuncles should receive prompt medical attention. The doctor may suggest the use of warm compresses, which help stimulate an adequate blood supply and bring an infected lesion to a head. Doctors usually treat carbuncles by lancing and draining the lesion and also prescribing an antibiotic. Parents should discard all soiled compresses or dressings to prevent possible infection of other family members.

Compare BOILS.

Cardiopulmonary resuscitation

A technique for reviving anyone whose heartbeat and breathing have suddenly stopped. Cardiopulmonary resuscitation (CPR) basically involves both mouth-to-mouth artificial respiration and closed-chest massage—exerting rhythmic pressure against the breastbone in an effort to stimulate the heart to contract.

Ideally, **UNTRAINED PERSONS SHOULD NOT PERFORM CPR.** Without a firm knowledge of correct CPR technique, a would-be Good Samaritan could do serious damage to a victim, including fractured ribs, punctured lungs, or direct injury to the heart. The technique cannot be learned from reading books or manuals; it requires personal instruction from an expert. Free courses in CPR techniques are conducted regularly throughout the United States. Parents are urged to take such a course; you could save your child's life or someone else's.

CPR must never be performed on an unconscious person

whose heart is still beating. The heartbeat can be determined by checking the pulse at a victim's wrist or, probably simpler for lay people, by checking whether the carotid arteries—along the sides of the neck—are beating. It is also essential to make sure a victim's air passages are clear. Any vomitus or secretions should be removed with the fingers or a handkerchief.

See also: CHOKING.

Celiac disease

See MALABSORPTION SYNDROME.

Chest deformity

See PIGEON CHEST, SUNKEN CHEST.

Chest pain

Magazines and other media have over the past several years given so much attention to the possibly dire implications of chest pain, parents should be reassured to know that in most instances chest pain in children and adolescents is most often perfectly harmless.

Adolescents are especially prone to recurrent episodes of sharp pain in the front of the chest, perhaps with a sensation of shortness of breath. There is no known cause for this; it's probably related to growth and activity.

Children's chest pain is often related to overeating, which causes INDIGESTION, or muscular strain from playing hard.

Unless the pain is prolonged, persistent, severe, or seems to limit activity, parents need not be too concerned.

See also: PLEURISY, PNEUMONIA, PNEUMOTHORAX.
Compare ABDOMINAL PAIN.

Chickenpox

A highly contagious infectious disease caused by a member of the herpes virus family called varicella, so that the disorder's technical name is varicella. Young infants up to about the age of six months are thought to possess natural immunity, although they may contract the disease in rare circumstances. Peak incidence occurs between the ages of five and nine, although older children and even adults can be infected—and from the age of ten onward the victim feels more ill.

The incubation period is about fourteen days, although it may range from eleven days to twenty, after which time separate spots begin to appear all over the body, sometimes even inside the cheeks, on the roof of the mouth, or in the scalp, although they tend to be concentrated mostly on the chest, back, and upper thighs. The spots appear in crops, beginning as small pink marks. Within just a few hours the spots turn into tiny blisters and look like drops of water resting on the skin. They vary in size from that of a pinhead to a split pea. Next the blisters cloud over and form a crust. Somewhere between ten and twenty days, the crust scabs fall away and leave pink marks. These marks eventually disappear entirely; parents can be reassured that scarring is rare.

The main discomfort of chickenpox comes from the itching. Relief is often possible with one of the orally administered medications prescribed by a doctor. It is important to keep the child from scratching or picking at the scabs—not, contrary to common belief, because it spreads the disease itself, which is viral and blood-borne, but because opening the skin may provide a route for infection by bacteria or do enough damage to scar the skin.

Younger children ill with chickenpox usually have just a slight fever at first; they rarely feel ill enough to remain in bed more than four or five days and need not remain in bed at all unless they feel badly enough. Children should be kept isolated for about one week after the rash appears; they are infectious only as long as new crops of lesions are developing. The contagious period ranges from one or two days before the rash appears to about five or six days after that time.

When the rash of chickenpox first appears, parents should tell the doctor so he or she can confirm the diagnosis and recommend appropriate itch-relieving medications that can be taken orally (for example, pediatric forms of Benadryl and Atarax). Cool baths will also help relieve itching. Chickenpox is essentially a home-treatable disease unless your child has leukemia or some other serious disorder that affects the body's immune system, in which case special medical attention is required to prevent serious side effects of this usually mild childhood illness. Parents should also be aware that there seems to be a connection between varicella and REYE'S SYNDROME. If a youngster, during the course of chickenpox or shortly thereafter, develops severe headaches, profuse vomiting, or abnormal behavior, then an urgent medical evaluation is advised.

Compare MEASLES.

Child abuse

The felony of physical assault, severe emotional abuse, and/or life-threatening neglect and deprivation seems to be on the rise. It is a particularly serious problem because many studies have shown that abused children, once they are grown up, tend to abuse their own children, thus perpetuating a cycle that is extremely damaging to everyone concerned, as well as to society at large.

Even seemingly minor episodes, such as reprimanding children by using cruel or frightening threats, humiliating them by teasing them in front of their friends or other family members, or further punishing them when they are already contrite, can create confusion and anxiety in developing minds. Parents who seem to have trouble in this area or who have cause to worry about their own bad tempers might help themselves and their children by discussing such issues with a physician or psychologist.

As to the serious and criminal offense that warrants the term *child abuse,* concerned parents may wish to know that an agency called The National Child Abuse Hotline (1-800-422-4453 or 1-800-4-A-CHILD, toll-free) now exists in the United States. The group guarantees anonymity to callers who wish to report abuse or suspected abuse. The report will be treated confidentially, and callers are protected from any liability in case a lawsuit should arise. The agency's sole aims are to stop child abuse and prevent further instances, and to help the parent who is fearful of potentially abusing his or her child.

Additional information on child abuse may be obtained by writing or calling the International Society for the Prevention of Child Abuse and Neglect, at 1205 Oneida Street, Denver, CO 80220, telephone (303) 321-3963.

Chills

An attack of shivering accompanied by the sensation of coldness. It typically precedes many fevers children get, and it may occur when youngsters are contracting influenza, pneumonia, or other infectious diseases. However, a chill is not always a symptom of infection; it may occur when a child has been given fever-reducing medications, including aspirin. Sometimes chills accompany an allergic reaction, a transfusion reaction, or the presence of some malignancy. Repeated chills are common in blood-carried infections caused by bacteria (bacteremia), in acute infections of the kidney, when the child has endocarditis (an inflammation of the membrane that lines the heart and its valves), and with certain abscesses.

Children experiencing chills should be made as comfortable as possible in a warm, but not stuffy, room, and perhaps by adding an extra blanket. Hot drinks may be soothing. Parents should take the child's temperature as soon as possible, repeating this about every twenty minutes until twenty minutes after the chill subsides. If the parent decides to seek medical advice, this temperature record, as well as information about the duration and severity of the chill, is helpful to the physician.

See also: COMMON COLD.

Choking

Intended for public dissemination, the following is the latest policy statement from the American Academy of Pediatrics.

First Aid for the Choking Child

The aspiration of a foreign body is a common hazard and the second greatest cause of home accidental death in children less than five years old. The National Safety Council reported more than 450 childhood deaths in 1978 caused by the accidental ingestion or inhalation of objects or foods resulting in the obstruction of respiratory passages.

Any foreign body in the upper airway is an immediate threat to life and requires urgent removal. If the child can speak or breathe and is coughing, any maneuvers are dangerous and unnecessary. If the choking child is unable to breathe or make a sound, turn the child's head and face down over your knees and forcefully give four back blows in an effort to propel the object from the windpipe. If this procedure fails, deliver four chest thrusts rapidly. Repeat these procedures as necessary if there is no response. Finger probing of the mouth should be attempted only if the foreign body is visualized. If the victim is an infant, place him over your forearm for the maneuvers. Older children can be placed on the rescuer's lap or on the floor.

Rapid transport to a medical facility is urgent if these first-aid measures fail.

See also: CARDIOPULMONARY RESUSCITATION, POISONING.

Chorea

A nervous disorder characterized by involuntary muscular twitching and irregular jerky movements.

Sydenham's chorea, also known as St. Vitus' dance, can occur as a complication of streptococcal infections and is sometimes associated with RHEUMATIC FEVER. A sedative or tranquilizer can be helpful in some cases, but the condition, more common in girls than in boys, usually subsides within about three months, or six to eight months at the most. Parents need not be unduly concerned, and children should be given plenty of reassurance that the condition is temporary and there will be no lasting physical effects and no damage to the mind.

A diagnosis of Huntington's chorea is far more serious. It is a hereditary disease that eventually leads to mental deterioration, although symptoms usually do not occur until victims are in their mid-thirties. However, the genetic possibility of transmission is so high that authorities advise members of any family with a known history of the disease not to have children.

Since people without medical training are not in a position

to assess children's twitching, clumsiness, or impaired muscular coordination, parents should take any child showing these symptoms to a doctor. In some instances children subconsciously or unconsciously display unusual arm, leg, or facial movements because of psychological stress.

Cigarette smoking

Despite governmental efforts to warn the public of the hazards of cigarette smoking, 80 percent of teenagers will experiment with cigarette smoking and some 20 to 30 percent will become regular smokers by age eighteen.

Media presentations depict smokers as self-assured, mature, and powerful figures. Since these are goals of adolescence, teenagers are particularly susceptible to such role models.

A directive not to smoke, whether stated before or after the fact, is unlikely to work, for rebellion and striving toward independence are natural events in the life of the teenager. A better tack might be emphasizing self-image—reminding the teenager that unpleasant odors will be on their clothes and breath, that skin yellows and wrinkles earlier in individuals who smoke, that yellow teeth and persistent coughing are unattractive, and that they may win even more respect from their peers if they can say no.

As the growing child becomes more aware of health issues, he or she may be more amenable to considering the long-term effects on health—changes in blood pressure and heart rate, the highly increased risk of contracting lung cancer or other lung diseases.

Circumcision

A surgical procedure in which the prepuce (the skin fold covering the head of the penis) is removed.

Except as a matter of religious ritual, circumcision is now the object of considerable controversy. Advocates stress ease of hygiene, avoidance of inflammation, and less risk of contracting venereal disease. The American Academy of Pediatrics claims there is no evidence to support *routine* performance of the operation. When an uncircumcised baby is bathed, the foreskin should be brought all the way back so that the head of the penis can be properly cleaned. As the little boy grows, he can be taught to do this himself.

When circumcision is performed, it is usually done shortly after birth. No anesthetic is used and the operation usually takes no more than fifteen minutes. Either a metal or plastic bell is used to control the bleeding while the skin is removed. In some techniques a plastic ring is left on to provide pressure so that no bleeding occurs and to help promote proper healing. This plastic device should fall off by the eighth day; if it doesn't, parents should contact the baby's doctor.

Care of a circumcision is relatively simple. For the first few days after the operation there may be a thick, yellow material that adheres as healing takes place. Merely keep the area well cleaned with soap and water and apply petroleum jelly to prevent irritation from diapers or other underclothing. If there is any untoward swelling, bleeding, or apparent difficulty in urinating, call the doctor.

On occasion an extra fold of skin will remain after circumcision. Just like the foreskin, this fold of skin should be retracted for washing.

Cloudy urine

See URINE AND URINATION.

Club foot

A congenital (present-at-birth) abnormality in which the heel is high and the foot and toes point downward and inward. It is not too common a disorder, occurring in somewhat less than 1 out of every 1000 births, and it is sometimes accompanied by other malformations (for example, lack of proper closure in the bony segments around the spinal cord). It is somewhat more common in males than in females, and may occur more frequently in the case of multiple births.

Treatment usually consists of applying a series of casts that are wedged in positions that will allow gradual movement of the foot back into its normal position. Later, corrective shoes are worn until the growth period ends. In less severe cases splinting may correct the abnormality, and in more severe cases surgical correction may be required. Prompt treatment is very important. If possible, it should begin right after birth as soon as the condition is noticed.

Cold

See COMMON COLD.

Cold sore

A cold sore is a localized infection caused by the herpes simplex virus, Type I (not the herpes virus that causes the venereal disease). It sometimes accompanies the common cold, is often recurrent, and characteristically develops into a small group of fever blisters, especially around the lips and at the corners of the mouth.

The discomfort of cold sores can sometimes be relieved by the application of skin balms, lotions, or glycerin-type preparations. Parents of children who suffer a prolonged bout of cold sores may wish to have a doctor check out the lesion to make sure it is not a bacterical infection such as impetigo.

See also: HERPES SIMPLEX.

Colic

A collection of symptoms and signs usually confined to very young infants. It does no permanent harm and almost always disappears of its own accord by the time the baby is three or four months old.

However, until that time the irritability of an infant in apparent pain may cause enormous physical and psychological stress to the parents, who often need to be reassured that they are not guilty of anything, that they are not being bad parents, and that the infant is not seriously ill and will recover. Sometimes a sympathetic physician will suggest that the colicky baby be placed in the hands of a competent temporary caretaker while the distraught parents enjoy a couple hours out at dinner or some distracting show or musical event.

The cause of colic is unknown, although some authorities believe it may be connected to one or more of the following: swallowing air, overfeeding, intestinal allergy, poor digestion in the form of excessive fermentation of carbohydrates in the intestines, and, on rare occasion, some emotional upset.

It is easy to understand parents' concern. The infant with colic may cry incessantly, apparently from ABDOMINAL PAIN. The abdomen is usually distended and tense, and colicky infants will typically draw up their legs against the abdomen and clench their hands. An attack, often occurring at about the same time each day, usually in late afternoon or evening, may last from two to about ten minutes, only to be followed by another one a very short time later. Sometimes an attack will subside only when the child is completely exhausted.

Parents can often help relieve colic attacks by placing the baby stomach-down across their knees or against the shoulder, or in the crib on a pillow, gently rubbing the baby's back. Sometimes placing a hot-water bottle filled with lukewarm water against the infant's stomach helps. Rectal stimulation with a lubricated thermometer or a glycerin suppository may be effective because it's been noticed that colicky babies seem to be relieved when they have a bowel movement or pass gas.

If the doctor suspects a MILK ALLERGY, a switch to soybean milk may be suggested. If the infant is being breast-fed, the mother may be asked to eliminate milk from her diet. In especially severe cases a physician may prescribe a sedative for the child.

If attacks of colic are associated with vomiting or abdominal bloating, it is particularly important to have the child examined medically to determine if something more serious, such as INTESTINAL OBSTRUCTION, may be causing the infant's pain.

Colitis

Simply defined, this disorder is an inflammation of the colon (the large intestine). Colitis may be attached to a wide range of underlying conditions, such as AMEBIC DYSENTERY and BACILLARY DYSENTERY.

Colitis is not particularly prevalent in childhood. Its highest incidence occurs between the ages of fifteen and forty. However, immediate medical attention is essential at the first suggestion of ulcerative colitis, as in severe, rapidly progressive first attacks the disease can be life threatening. In addition to inflammation, ulcerative colitis involves ulceration of the mucous membrane that lines the large intestine. The condition is marked by acute ABDOMINAL PAIN and the frequent passage of foul-smelling, watery stools that contain blood, mucus, and pus. Sometimes the disease begins with a sudden and violent attack of bloody DIARRHEA and high fever of 103° to 104°F.

Collapsed lung

See PNEUMOTHORAX.

Combative behavior

See AGGRESSIVE BEHAVIOR.

Common cold

Viruses, the smallest particles capable of causing disease, are responsible for the common cold. A cold can be caused by any one of more than a hundred different viruses, which is why many children, and adults, seem to have a cold that lasts all winter; they suffer from one infection after another.

Colds are spread by the viruses simply floating through the air from one child's nose and mouth to another child's nose and mouth. Crowding indoors, such as in day-care and school settings, makes infection almost impossible to avoid. The frequency of colds in young children probably builds future immunity. This explains why young children can normally be expected to get up to eight colds each year, while adolescents average only two to four per year.

Symptoms usually include chills, sore throat, runny nose, stuffy nose (nasal congestion), slight headache, and, sometimes, a cough and fever. Colds usually last from three to seven days. Since viruses do not respond to antibiotics or to other drugs that fight bacteria, treatment remains geared to relieving discomfort and being prudent about exposing others to the cold virus. Keep the child home at least three days—the contagious period. A humidifier may relieve the congestion and coughing that is often particularly bad at night. Infants can be placed on their bellies to improve nasal drainage. Drinking lots of liquid will help thin mucous secretions, but older children should cut back on milk, which tends to thicken these secretions. When parents give the child nonprescription drugs such as aspirinlike compounds, nose drops or sprays, or preparations that soothe throats and lessen coughing, always follow label directions carefully.

Normally the child will not need a doctor's evaluation unless there are complications, for example: a persisting temperature of over 102°F; a cough that produces thick, discolored material; swollen glands; pain in the teeth or a severe headache; discoloring of the nails, skin, or lips; and any marked change in the child's normal behavior pattern. On occasion a bad cold may lead to SINUSITIS (inflammation of the sinuses), EAR INFECTION, or BRONCHITIS.

Compulsive behavior

A form of behavior in which there is repetition of a particular physical act or acts over a long period of time. It seems to be more common in young school-age children.

Children may, for example, be able to go to sleep only after every pair of socks in the bedroom is carefully rolled and placed in rows in a dresser drawer. A classic example is the need to wash one's hands twenty or thirty times a day when there is no reason to do so.

Often such actions are performed as substitutes for thinking about frightening, tension-causing feelings of anger or resentment, or as a means of avoiding some underlying conflict. The compulsive behavior, being ritualistic, affords the child some magic way of warding off thoughts and feelings he or she senses it is best to keep on an unconscious level. If these acts are severe enough to interfere with normal functioning, or if they seem to be preventing a child from developing new social skills normal for school-age youngsters, parents are advised to seek help from a physician or psychologist.

On the other hand, normal school-age children frequently develop temporary behavior patterns that seem ritualistic and obsessive. For example, they may avoid stepping on cracks in the sidewalk; tell endless jokes that seem nonsensical to adults; make noises with their tongues; annoy adults by counting telephone poles or reading signs out loud during automobile trips; cross their eyes for the fun of it; or, sometimes, even develop little facial tics (repetitive muscle spasms) that distort their features and alarm concerned parents. For the most part, these behaviors reflect youngsters' attempts to master their own bodies and put the environment into some ordered relationship.

Parents should grin and bear it and not rush the child off for counseling or a neurological examination unless the behavior persists unduly or unless a young adolescent suddenly exhibits compulsive behavior that is quite different in nature and intensity from his or her usual patterns.

Concussion

A violent jarring of the brain, a cerebral concussion, caused by a blow to the head or a HEAD INJURY such as might occur when a child falls and becomes unconscious. The trauma may seem insignificant, but the damage may be severe. Dizziness, headaches, and vomiting may be dominant symptoms of concussion.

Return of full consciousness is gradual, although it usually takes only a few minutes. Parents used to be advised to keep the child awake, but it is now considered sufficient to awaken concussion victims every two hours to check for the signs described below.

Whenever parents have the slightest cause to suspect that a child has sustained a concussion, or if the child has been unconscious even briefly, they should notify a doctor immediately. Prompt medical evaluation and perhaps X rays will be needed to ensure that there is no skull fracture or any rupture of blood vessels within the brain.

Hospitalization may or may not be necessary; it depends on the results of the physician's neurological examination. If the child soon regains normal alertness, doctors have discovered no signs or symptoms of potentially serious brain damage, and the parents can be counted on to be watchful, the youngster may be allowed to go home.

Parents should remain alert to the signs listed below that

may follow a concussion. If they occur, the doctor should be notified immediately or the child should be taken for emergency medical assessment.

1. Nonuse of an arm or leg
2. Convulsions
3. Inequality in the size of the pupils of the eyes
4. Repeated vomiting
5. Unusual behavior
6. Difficulty in arousing the child

Each of these abnormalities should be especially checked for every two hours when the child is awakened during the night.

Confusion

See DISORIENTATION.

Conjunctivitis

Commonly called pinkeye, this condition is an inflammation of the conjunctiva (the membrane that lines the eyelid and covers the white of the eye). In a newborn it may occur because of the infant's reaction to silver nitrate, a chemical instilled at the time of delivery. In rare instances a newborn infant's conjunctivitis may occur because silver nitrate is *not* instilled and the mother has gonorrhea. Less infrequently, the condition may be a reaction to specks of dirt or other foreign objects. By far the most common cause of pinkeye is bacterial or viral infections that are highly contagious and seem to appear in epidemics.

The first signs of conjunctivitis are usually a burning or smarting sensation of the eyelids, along with intense itching. The white of the eye becomes pink or bright red, and the eye waters excessively. This watery discharge may change to a sticky secretion containing pus, which causes the eyelashes and eyelids to stick together, especially when the child sleeps. The lids often become swollen, and in severe cases both eyes are involved.

Mild forms of pinkeye usually clear up within a few days, especially if the outsides of the eyes are gently and regularly bathed in warm water that has been previously boiled to kill any germs that may have been present in it. Parents can soak a cotton ball in the water and then hold it against the child's closed eye for about ten minutes. This should be repeated several times throughout the day and just before the child goes to bed.

If the parent seeks medical advice and the doctor has prescribed an antibiotic ointment, be careful to apply the medication correctly. An ointment is spread in a thin line along the lower eyelid, which is retracted (held down). Use of eyedrops is often restricted to older children because of difficulties the most dedicated parent may experience when trying to instill drops into a squirming youngster's eye.

When pinkeye is severe or tends to recur frequently, the child should be examined and treated by a doctor.

Constipation

The difficult and too-infrequent passage of dry, hard bowel movements.

In infants constipation may result from drinking too much milk. Diet is also an important factor in youngsters and older children, especially if they eat too little fiber or roughage. Sometimes children will repeatedly fail to heed the "call of nature"; when this happens the sensation of having to pass stools will disappear for a while. The result is that waste products of digestion continue to accumulate in the rectum (lower end of the large intestine), where they become large and hardened and increasingly difficult to pass. Especially in older children and adolescents, chronic constipation is sometimes related to excessive worry, anxiety, fear, or other forms of emotional tension. Frequent use of laxatives, as well as certain drugs, such as intestinal antispasmodics, that inhibit normal motion of the bowels can also cause constipation. Some cases of constipation are due to lack of fluid intake, since fluids help keep the stools soft.

Harsh laxatives should not be given to children. Indeed, any laxative should be given only with considerable caution. Be sure to follow label instructions for children's doses, and be sure never to exceed that dosage or extend the time limits that are noted. Mineral oil is a fairly safe means of softening the stools in children who are constipated; it also helps reduce straining during bowel movements. For children from about two to five years of age, the usual dosage is one tablespoonful in the morning and at night. This may be continued until loose or normal bowel movements occur on a daily basis. Commercial stool softeners can also be used to keep the bowel movements at a proper consistency, and infants can usually obtain prompt relief when their rectums are stimulated by a glycerin suppository.

If improvement isn't noted within three days, or if a child suffers over a prolonged period from repeated bouts of constipation, parents should consult a doctor. Should ABDOMINAL PAIN be one of the symptoms of constipation, the child should also be taken to a doctor (not necessarily an urgent situation) in case there is a more complex problem that requires diagnosis and treatment.

Finally, parents should understand that for some children, just as in adults, having bowel movements only about three or four times a week is a normal pattern. So in many ways it is the degree of change from children's usual elimination pattern that signals constipation or diarrhea.

Compare DIARRHEA.

Convulsions

Abnormal muscle contractions, often of a violent nature, in which the child jerks and twists in an uncontrolled fashion. There is a loss of consciousness and there may be a loss of control of urine flow or bowel movements. Often there is a gurgling in the throat and an upward rolling of the eyes.

Parents should be reassured that not all convulsions indicate serious problems. Young children, particularly toddlers, may suffer convulsions as a result of sudden, rapid rises in body temperature.

On the other hand, convulsions may occur as a result of serious infections such as MENINGITIS or ENCEPHALITIS; because of a lack of oxygen or HYPOGLYCEMIA (extremely low blood sugar); or from a seizure disorder.

Whatever the cause and however brief the episode, a child having convulsions is extremely upsetting to parents who witness these contortions and feel helpless. Remaining calm is a *must.* Make no attempt to restrain the twitching, and do not move the child. However, any hard objects in the area should be removed and something soft, like a pillow, can be placed under the child's head. If the convulsions seem severe enough that the child might accidentally bite his or her own tongue, parents can wrap some long piece of fairly hard material, such as a stick, in a handkerchief or other piece of handy fabric and place it between the child's teeth.

People are often advised to make sure that the airway is not blocked, but if the child's teeth are tightly clenched, this may not be possible. Should vomiting occur, turn the child's head sideways so the vomitus drains outward and doesn't cause choking. As soon as the jerking or twisting stops, the child should be wrapped warmly and taken to a doctor or medical facility. A thorough medical evaluation is necessary to determine the cause of the convulsive seizure and plan any necessary treatment.

See also: FEVER CONVULSION.

Convulsive disorders

See SEIZURE DISORDERS.

Cord drainage

See UMBILICAL CORD.

Cough

A reflexive action by which the body attempts to clear the airway or lungs of a secretion, foreign body, or irritation.

By far the commonest cause of children's coughing is acute respiratory infection, including the common cold. Infants under eighteen months old are susceptible to a viral illness called BRONCHIOLITIS, in which first coughing and then wheezing are prominent symptoms and the baby breathes rapidly. When children appear to be quite ill and their temperature is high (above 102° or 103°F), PNEUMONIA may be suspected. The cough in BRONCHITIS is particularly harsh sounding, and that of PERTUSSIS (whooping cough) is accompanied by a characteristic whooping sound from the throat. ALLERGIES and ASTHMA are notorious causes of children's recurrent and persistent coughs.

With the possible exception of the minor cough of the common cold, parents should check with a physician. Any of the diseases noted warrant medical attention, as does any cough that lasts more than three or four days or is associated with other signs or symptoms, for example, a temperature of over 101°F, or shortness of breath, or, of course, when blood-tinged secretions are found in material a child coughs up. Sometimes this represents nothing more than the bursting of tiny blood capillaries from the strain of coughing, but a parent should verify this with a doctor.

The minor cough of a simple cold can be relieved by over-the-counter preparations, use of a vaporizer, and giving the child plenty of liquids to keep secretions watery and flowing.

CPR

See CARDIOPULMONARY RESUSCITATION.

Cradle cap

The popular term for a kind of skin inflammation, a seborrheic dermatitis, that sometimes occurs in infants between birth and six months, usually clearing up by the time they are a year old. It is generally most prominent on the scalp, although sometimes other areas, such as the eyebrows, ears, armpits, and diaper areas, are affected. Thick, yellowish, scaly crusts appear over the affected area(s).

The application of baby oil only aggravates the condition, since it is caused by a buildup of natural body oils. Milder cases can often be controlled simply by vigorously washing the scalp with soap and water, then gently scraping away all the scales with a very soft brush or very fine toothed comb. Parents need not be afraid of damaging the fontanel (soft spot); the area is pliable but dense, and the pressure of a good shampooing will do no damage.

In more persistent cases the child's physician may prescribe a corticosteroid preparation or a sulfur ointment in addition to a special medicated shampoo. Once the scalp condition clears, any associated body rashes also clear up.

Cretinism

See THYROID DISORDERS.

Crib death

See SUDDEN INFANT DEATH SYNDROME.

Cross-dressing

See TRANSVESTISM.

Cross-eye

See STRABISMUS.

Croup

A general term that describes a distinctly resonant, barking cough usually accompanied by difficulty in breathing and hoarseness. It occurs when there is a spasm or obstruction of the larynx (the voice box). Most often it is caused by an acute viral infection of the upper and lower parts of the respiratory tract; but it may also occur as a complication of LARYNGITIS, PERTUSSIS (whooping cough), or DIPHTHERIA, or because of an allergy or the presence of a foreign body in the larynx.

Children from about three months to seven years are most susceptible to croup, and the malady usually strikes during winter months.

In most instances croup presents no real threat, even though an attack may be as alarming to the parents as to the child. Usually these children have colds. They wake up at night because a trickle of mucus or other discharge has irritated and blocked the larynx, causing it to go into a brief spasm. This temporarily interferes with normal breathing and the child has a violent attack of coughing. The hoarse cough and the sudden wakening with a breathing difficulty are frightening. The fright may cause the spasms to worsen. If parents panic, the situation tends to worsen. Gentle reassurance and perhaps a cup of cocoa or some other drink that is special to the child can ease the child's anxiety. A good way to assess severity is to note whether the child is croupy only when coughing or whether noisy breathing continues when the child is resting. If the noise continues, the child should be seen by a doctor.

Croup caused by viral infection may last up to a week. Children should be kept comfortable and given plenty to drink. Home treatment can be provided by using cold-steam humidifiers or steam from a hot tub or shower. The parent should stay with the child as the bathroom door is shut to allow steam to accumulate. Periods of exposure to the steam should be limited to ten minutes. If the croup is not relieved by steam inhalation, medical attention should be sought.

Particularly in very small children, marked respiratory distress or other problems may require hospitalization so that these children can be under constant observation and be given oxygen. In severe cases the air passages may become obstructed and a tracheotomy (cutting a temporary air passage into the throat) may be necessary.

An extremely severe and dangerous form of croup is called epiglottitis. The child with this disease very rapidly develops difficulty breathing, perhaps even turning blue in a matter of a few hours. High fever is present and the child looks very ill. Swallowing is so painful that children with epiglottitis cannot swallow their own saliva, so they drool. They also want to sit upright, leaning forward as a natural defense against complete closure of the airway. The child with severe croup needs immediate emergency medical attention.

Crying

A common physical reaction of infants and children. As parents well know, it can indicate pain, fear, frustration, or a physical need. The subject is mentioned here mainly because of the tendency adults have of constantly telling a child *not* to cry.

An infant cries for a very basic reason: he or she has no other method of complaining verbally. Within the child's first weeks of life parents usually learn to differentiate the pitch and volume used when infants are hungry, uncomfortable, afraid, tired, and so on.

As the child learns to talk, crying is still used as an emotional release. Even adults say, "I felt better after I had a good cry." Rather than eliminating the crying, parents should try to find out what's causing the child to cry. Often simple reassurance is all that is needed.

See also: IRRITABILITY.

Cuts

Small cuts, technically known as lacerations, of the child's skin need little attention other than what common sense dictates: exert pressure to stop the bleeding; clean the wound with soap and water and apply a nonstick dressing. Small cuts heal with little, if any, scarring.

If the edges of the wound are widely separated, use bandage strips to draw them together. If that does not work, suturing (stitching) by a physician may be required.

The wound should be observed for spreading redness or any drainage of pus, which might indicate an infection that requires medical attention.

Parents should keep a record of their children's immunization against tetanus. For a clean, uncontaminated wound, a tetanus booster within the last ten years should suffice. For a dirty wound—say, from rusty nails or when there's been exposure to contaminated materials—the child should have had a tetanus booster shot within the last five years. If there's any doubt, contact the child's doctor.

Larger wounds, especially on the face, may leave prominent scars. It may take two years before facial scars stabilize. Careful suturing by a qualified surgeon may minimize or even eliminate such scars.

Cyanosis

Blueness of the skin, mucous membranes, and nail beds caused by an inadequate amount of oxygen in the circulating blood. The skin may also appear slightly grayish or slatelike in color.

Prompt medical attention is essential to discover the underlying cause and to avoid life-threatening complications. Congenital (present-at-birth) cyanosis may be associated with various kinds of defects in the heart or lungs. Surgical or other medical procedures are usually successful in correcting the condition.

Cystic fibrosis

An inherited disease occurring in about 1 in 2000 live births, in Caucasian children.

The exact cause is unknown, but it affects glands that secrete by means of ducts. Thick secretions clog mucous glands lining the respiratory tract. These thick, mucouslike secretions also obstruct the pancreas duct system so that enzymes necessary for proper digestion and absorption fail to operate. Sweat glands also malfunction.

Cystic fibrosis usually begins in infancy. The child tends to have chronic respiratory infections and a lack of tolerance for heat; excessive sweating is common. Occasionally there is an obstruction of the small intestine during the first few days of life because of thick greenish meconium (a substance created in the baby's intestinal tract while the infant is in the uterus).

By the age of about one year, about 80 percent of children affected will show disturbances in breathing or digestion. Cough is the most troublesome symptom during the early stages of the disease, and at first it may be mistaken for whooping cough. Episodes of vomiting also occur. Older infants and children will have steatorrhea (excessive amounts of fat in bowel movements). Older children may sweat profusely, which can lead to a severe loss of essential body fluids and salts. Unless this situation is corrected by appropriate therapy, the child may suffer DEHYDRATION and circulatory failure.

Some sufferers survive into adulthood in spite of the recurrent infections. There is no known cure for the disease. However, aggressive medical treatment can offer the child some relief through drainage of pus-filled mucous secretions from the respiratory tract; the use of pancreatic enzymes to help the gastrointestinal tract digest nutrients; antibiotics to ward off lung infections; and supervised vitamin therapy.

Professional help can also be extended to the parents, who may want genetic counseling about having other children as well as assistance in dealing with the fact that their child has a fatal disease. Additional information about these matters and about the disease itself can be obtained from the Cystic Fibrosis Foundation.

Cystitis

An inflammation of the urinary bladder, usually caused by a bacterial infection. Although it is not a common disease of childhood, it tends to occur somewhat more often in girls, because the female urethra (the passageway leading from the bladder to the outside opening) is much shorter than in males and provides easier access for infectious organisms.

The disease may be acute or chronic. In the acute form the young person will typically complain of painful urination and the frequent urge to pass urine even though the bladder may be empty. Freshly passed urine is clouded in appearance, because of the presence of pus, and often has a strong, fishy odor. A steady dull ache may be experienced in the lower part of the abdomen, which is quite sensitive to the slightest pressure. Sometimes the urethra is also inflamed (urethritis), and in severe forms of cystitis the patient may have a high fever (102°F) and sweat profusely.

The diagnosis is confirmed by laboratory tests involving bacterial counts in the urine. Other tests such as X rays are used to make sure the infection is not related to a structural defect or obstruction of the urinary system. The doctor must also make sure that the infection is, in fact, restricted to the bladder and has not spread upward to the kidneys. Sometimes a urologist (a doctor specializing in disease of the urinary system) will use a special instrument called a cystoscope to inspect the inside of the urethra and bladder.

Successful treatment involves the early administration of an appropriate antibiotic, drinking lots of water and other fluids, and restricting intake of spicy foods or other substances that might irritate the bladder after they are filtered to become part of the urine. Follow-up bacterial counts are usually taken to confirm recovery.

D

Deafness

Complete or partial loss of the ability to hear in one or both ears. It may be caused by any one of several factors, including infection, and the HEARING LOSS may be only temporary (as rarely occurs with too much earwax) or permanent (as in congenital deafness).

There are two basic classifications: *conductive deafness* and *nerve deafness.* Conductive deafness occurs when there is any interference with sound vibrations during their passage to the inner ear. In the outer passage; this interference could be caused by an infection that discharges obstructive fluid; swelling and closure of the passage; or, less commonly, by excessive earwax. In the so-called middle ear, inflammation or an obstructing growth of tissue or bone could cause deafness. Enlargement of a child's adenoids or similar lymph tissue at the back of the throat can block the opening of the eustachian tube (a short canal that connects this region with the middle ear); this blockage disturbs air pressure and reduces hearing. Rupture, inflammation, or scarring can affect the eardrum itself.

Nerve deafness, sometimes called perceptive deafness, is the most common cause of total and permanent deafness. It sometimes is a complication of some disease or injury that affects the cochlea (where sound vibrations are transformed into nerve impulses) or the auditory nerve (which transmits impulses to the brain).

Congenital deafness (deafness present from birth) is a rather rare condition for which the cause often remains unknown. Sometimes it may be connected to the mother having had rubella (German measles) during early pregnancy.

Observant parents will note very early on if their child is not responding to speech, the clapping of hands, sudden noises, and normal household noises. A newborn infant will show the "startle response" to a sudden, loud noise, and infants as young as three months can be tested by sophisticated audiometric (hearing-measuring) techniques. Parents who suspect some deficiency can, by the time their child is six to eight months old, try clapping their hands behind the child's head where he or she cannot see the action. This is important because sometimes a youngster learns to interpret the movements and gestures of the parents to compensate for unheard speech. Thus deafness can sometimes go undetected for two or three years—although if by that time the child is not speaking at least a few words that are correct and distinctly pronounced, parents should be suspicious, since deaf children cannot learn to imitate speech they don't hear.

Early medical evaluation is essential, for if children are not properly diagnosed and, when possible, treated, they may suffer irreparable psychological damage from being categorized by their age peers, schoolmates, teachers, and others as being slow, dumb, or stupid. Sometimes the removal of hardened and impacted ear wax is all that is needed. Various types of hearing aids (body aids, eyeglass aids, aids in the ear itself) can sometimes be used as early as the age of nine months. Many kinds of conduction deafness can be corrected surgically. If the child suffers permanent nerve deafness, he or she will need special training that teaches one to capitalize on other senses that are intact.

Death of parent or sibling

As is true of many aspects of children's behavior, reactions to traumatic events will be modeled on what surrounding adults do.

In the tragic events of a parent's or sibling's death, the survivors might best serve themselves and the child by *not* keeping a stiff upper lip. If the child is allowed to grieve openly and discuss feelings of loss, he or she may avoid or at least minimize the psychological problems that loss can incur. It is especially important that children be helped to understand that no matter what their secret moments of hate or wishing the person would go away, they are not guilty of killing their mother, father, sister, or brother.

On the other hand, the child should not be given special privileges, in the sense of permitting behavior that was not previously acceptable or the formation of an artificially close bond in vain efforts to make up for the loss. If symptoms of DEPRESSION develop, it may be helpful to enlist a professional who can assist the child in putting the death into a more appropriate perspective.

Dehydration

A physical state in which the total amount of water in the body is below what is needed to carry on normal metabolic (energy-exchanging) functions.

Dehydration is not uncommon in infants and small children who are given to frequent bouts of diarrhea or vomiting, which cause fluid loss. This, in turn, impairs the conduction of ions (small charged particles) that normally cause electric activity involved in the exchange of gases and solids that gives bodily parts the energy to do their jobs.

All this activity is a part of what is called metabolism. Infants have a metabolic rate that is as much as three times higher than that of adults. Therefore their fluid turnover is considerably faster, and dehydration can be a real threat to survival.

An affected infant or young child will become irritable, then lethargic, and a fever may develop. Parents may note the child's decreased frequency and quantity of urination. In more severe cases there may be loss of weight, skin dryness, and, in young infants, a kind of sinking of the fontanel or soft spot.

Real dehydration—as opposed to a very mild condition that makes children thirsty, and which parents can correct by giving lots of fluids by mouth—demands medical attention. Sometimes the lost water and salts can be replaced by oral solutions. Usually doctors will need to assess the severity of the dehydration and decide on a course of treatment that most likely includes replacement of lost body fluids through the intravenous administration of special solutions.

Depression

An emotional state characterized by an intense feeling of sadness, believed to occur because of feelings of loss or lack of love, although chemical imbalances may cause what is termed *biologic depression.*

Depression was formerly thought to be basically an adult disease, but experts in the field now realize that it is not so rare in children, especially school-age children and adolescents. Even infants can feel sad, which is usually signaled by poor weight gain and a general lack of response to the environment.

Parents should be particularly aware of BEHAVIOR CHANGES in the child. They may note symptoms such as sleep disturbances, tearfulness, poor appetite, and low energy levels. There may be a withdrawal from social activities or a faltering academic performance in school. Sometimes other behaviors, such as anxiety reactions, aggressive behavior, temper tantrum, hyperactivity, restless behavior, complaints of headache or abdominal pain, or just plain misbehavior or constant clowning around may mask the depressive state. Eventually, the feelings may become so intense that they interfere with the child's day-to-day activities; personal hygiene or doing simple everyday tasks may suffer. When such changes occur, it is best not to punish the child; neither is it appropriate to try to encourage an unrealistic sense of optimism. If parents cannot understand what is going on and cannot help their depressed children talk out the depression and work it through, and a physician can find no biological basis for the depression, it is definitely advisable to seek a professional psychological evaluation. This is, of course, mandatory should the young person be preoccupied with thoughts about death or SUICIDE. Parents should be particularly sensitive to a depressed adolescent suddenly becoming overly joyful; sometimes this signals a resolve to commit suicide.

Dermatitis

Any inflammation of the skin caused by an infection, allergy, or contact with an irritative substance.

Destructive behavior

A form of behavior in which a child takes special pains to destroy physical objects such as toys. It is a type of AGGRESSIVE BEHAVIOR, but rather than directing anger toward other people (including playmates) or himself/herself, the child attacks inanimate objects. It should be distinguished from activities in which children do, quite normally, take things apart out of sheer curiosity. However, the behavior should be observed carefully for frequency and intensity, for often it is what psychologists and psychiatrists call displacement. That is, the child may well wish to destroy a playmate, sibling, or parent but "displaces" the anger onto inanimate objects. If destructiveness is the rule rather than the exception, parents may wish to seek professional assistance.

Diabetes mellitus

A disorder associated with a faulty metabolism of carbohydrates, usually because certain cells in the pancreas, called the islets of Langerhans, fail to secrete enough insulin. Insulin, circulated in the blood, is a hormone that regulates sugar metabolism. Exactly what causes this malfunction still remains unknown, but authorities have considerable evidence to indicate that the disease is hereditary.

Approximately 40 in every 10,000 children have diabetes mellitus. Unlike adults, who often experience a gradual onset after many years of a prediabetic condition, children often manifest the disease rather suddenly and often more severely. Early signs include weight loss; frequent passing of urine; an almost unquenchable thirst and hunger; itchy, dry skin; as well as weakness and fatigue. Later, additional symptoms often include difficulty in breathing, extreme fatigue, and gastrointestinal problems such as loss of appetite, abdominal pain, and vomiting.

If the child remains untreated, the gradual accumulation of sugar in the blood may result in what is known as a diabetic coma. In such a state the child loses consciousness and may not survive without prompt medical or first-aid treatment. Warning signs may include nausea (often followed by vomiting), drowsiness, dry mouth, and deepened breathing before the child passes out. The situation can be confused with coma or state of shock brought on by HYPOGLYCEMIA (too low a level of blood sugar), which sometimes occurs when an overdose of insulin too suddenly depletes the blood-sugar level.

Early medical assessment is needed so that appropriate treatment can be started with the diabetic child. A simple urine test may show glycosuria (too much sugar, in the form of glucose, in the urine). Blood samples may also be taken to see how well the patient tolerates glucose.

Sometimes chemicals called ketones will be present, and they often give a child's breath and urine a sweet, almost "sickeningly sweet," smell.

In most cases children with diabetes are treated with daily injections of insulin. If the child is old enough, he or she is instructed how to administer these shots and how to do finger-stick blood tests so that the child can adjust the daily dose if the need arises. Younger children's parents will be given the same instructions.

In the past diabetic children were advised to restrict sugar, starch, and other carbohydrates. However, most doctors now contend that, within reason, the child should be allowed to eat what the family eats. This may be particularly so with adolescents, who are apt to regard strict dietary rules as yet another interference with their growing independence—and one they are especially apt to ignore.

Heavy exercise tends to decrease the blood sugar level, so children hard at play may require less insulin than usual. All diabetic patients should carry with them an emergency supply of sugar to take when they sense that their blood-sugar level is falling. The symptoms are restlessness, confusion, faintness, cold perspiration, hunger, and muscular unsteadiness. It is a good idea for the child's friends to know about the crisis that can occur in diabetes, so that they, as well as the family, can help monitor signs and symptoms of lowered blood sugar levels.

Diabetic children should be checked frequently by their doctor, as a number of complications can occur. Checkups should include periodic eye examinations to prevent a condition known as diabetic retinopathy, where ruptured blood vessels can cause a swelling of the retina and gradual loss of vision.

With modern forms of treatment, the lives of diabetics are far less restricted and confining than they once were. Careful home monitoring of sugar levels will prevent later development of complications affecting organs such as the kidneys or eyes. To the extent that the doctor allows, parents should try not to be overprotective. Otherwise children with diabetes may develop emotional blocks about their own capacity to compete, have fun, and live lives that are essentially normal except for daily medication, keeping tabs on their condition, and seeing doctors more frequently than many people do.

Diaper rash

A term describing a group of red, inflamed rashes that at one time or another affect the bottoms of just about all infants and small children who wear diapers. In the commonest type of rash the skin appears reddened or even raw. It is most noticeable on the child's buttocks, abdomen, and inner thighs.

The most consistent reason for these rashes is the simple mechanical action of the wetness—from perspiration, urine, or stool—combined with the friction diapers make as the baby moves. Many culprits have been named: bacteria and funguses; ammonia content of urine; chemicals found in soaps, detergents, and disposable diapers. Sometimes the baby's doctor prescribes a special ointment, most especially if a yeast rash is caused by *Candida albicans.* It is impossible to control all the factors that may cause diaper rash. Also, most diaper rashes clear up spontaneously and do not require any heroic measures on the part of the parents or doctor.

Gentle cleansing with cotton and mild soap, followed by thorough drying, is important. When the diaper can be left off completely, there will be less moisture to contend with. At night the baby can sleep on a pile of diapers; this should leave much of the area free of wetness. When diapers are used, they should be loose-fitting cotton and worn without plastic overpants until the rash has cleared.

Once the rash is better, disposable diapers or plastic pants can be used again. Heavy talcum powders should be avoided because they increase friction. Dusting powders, including the medicated ones, may be helpful, and a topical cortisone cream greatly reduces inflammation. As with all medications, read and follow label instructions carefully.

If there are open, weeping spots, parents can apply compresses of salt solution: one level teaspoonful of salt to a pint of water that has been boiled, then cooled to room temperature. The compressing can be done four times a day for ten minutes each time.

Once the skin is broken, a bacterial or fungal infection can set in. Newborns are especially susceptible to staphylococcal infections that show as small pus-filled eruptions with bright red bases. A bright red rash with small, pinpoint-size red spots around the margin may indicate a yeast, which will require prescription medication. If signs such as these occur or the diaper rash fails to clear within three or four days, the child should be checked by a doctor so that an accurate diagnosis and an effective treatment can be made.

Diarrhea

A condition in which the BOWEL MOVEMENTS are abnormally frequent (more than six in twenty-four hours) and consist of loose and watery stools. The diagnosis also applies to less frequent stools that are "explosive" and unusually voluminous. Diarrhea occurs fairly frequently in babies and very young children, especially in its milder forms. Causes include overfeeding; eating foods, including milk, to which the child is especially sensitive; or a digestive-tract infection. Especially in babies, diarrhea may accompany some other feverish illness, a sore throat, or an ear infection. Older children and adolescents may sometimes suffer from diarrhea caused by nervous excitement before examinations in school or social events.

In its more severe form, childhood diarrhea may feature stools mixed with slight traces of blood or pus. When this happens the child's doctor must be consulted immediately so that the cause can be determined and appropriate treatment begun. Serious diarrhea in infants is especially dangerous because of the possibility of DEHYDRATION.

Parents should become concerned if the number of stools exceeds six or eight, especially if vomiting is present. Changes in activity, dry lips and mouth, and decreased frequency of urination are also signs that the infant or child may be developing problems.

See also: AMEBIC DYSENTERY, BACILLARY DYSENTERY, COLITIS, DEHYDRATION.
Compare CONSTIPATION.

Diet

For the first six to eight months of life, milk is the infant's main food. Special formulas can be used if mothers cannot or do not wish to breast-feed. New mothers can obtain useful information from their child's doctor about the best times and ways to add solid foods to the baby's diet. Children differ, and there is no set rule about what foods need be added and when. It is generally agreed that the child's own appetite will gradually lead to seeking a balanced diet, especially when a variety of nutritious and wholesome choices is offered. If a new taste is refused, don't force the child to eat the food. Wait until he or she is a little older before reintroducing the taste. Babies differ in their acceptance of new flavors and textures, and in Western culture almost all youngsters initially dislike highly spiced foods or unusually strong flavors.

In order to build a strong and healthy body, the child needs adequate amounts of carbohydrates, proteins, fats, minerals, and VITAMINS. Precisely how much is difficult to say. Often it is a matter of common sense: If the young child is thriving, attaining normal rates of growth, and appears strong and healthy, he or she is probably getting a diet that is adequate in essential nutrients. There is some controversy concerning vitamins; some doctors recommend vitamin supplements until a child is about two years old, after which time it is assumed that a well-balanced diet provides ample amounts. Other practitioners disagree. They hold that because of extensive processing, foods that Americans eat rarely provide optimal amounts of vitamins and minerals. Another problem may arise with the common use of preservatives in commercial foods. Some of these chemical additives have been tied to the development of serious diseases, so, on the whole, parents are best serving their children's needs when they serve fresh foods or ones that are not packaged with chemicals intended to keep them from spoiling.

Children's stomachs are small. They should not be expected to consume huge quantities of food; in fact, they should be discouraged from doing so because of digestive difficulties that may ensue. It is because of their small stomachs that children often prefer snacking to formal meals. Snacking is entirely appropriate, provided junk foods are avoided and the snacking isn't done too close to mealtime. Meals should be shared with the rest of the family. The child learns good table manners and gradually comes to enjoy mealtime conversations and the unhurried, peaceful atmosphere of sitting down to a good dinner. It is definitely *not* a time for arguing, coaxing, or forcing children to eat. Meals should be a pleasant occasion; if they are presented that way, they will gradually lure older children from overindulging in between-meal snacks as they grow to regard dinner as something to look forward to.

Nutritional problems in school-age children often come from skipping breakfast and eating unnutritious lunches. The latter may be a particular problem for children whose schools do not provide supervised lunches and who may spend lunch money on sweets or junk food. In adolescents, the opposite problem may occur. Suddenly concerned with their appearance and their attractiveness to members of the opposite sex, both girls and boys may put themselves on fad or crash diets that make exaggerated weight-loss claims. Parents should express sympathetic concern and reassure their child that the chunkiness somewhat common to the early teenage years will disappear as the young person grows and altered metabolism catches up with itself. Of course, when an adolescent is truly obese, parents should consider a medical consultation and the possibility of the child's undertaking a supervised program such as some of the professionally run summer camps devoted to weight loss.

About sweets: again, common sense is the key. Prohibiting a toddler, child, or adolescent any sweets will be regarded for what it is: cruel and unusual punishment. On the other hand, overindulgence in candies, sundae toppings, and other sugary treats can lead to bad teeth, probable nutritional imbalances, and the possibility of aggravating some medical problem such as a prediabetic condition. One method of discouraging the overindulgence of sweets is to see that healthy snack foods such as carrots, celery, apples, and cheese, etc., are commonly munched on at home. If parents sit around devouring boxes of chocolates, the child can hardly be expected to develop a preference for health-promoting snack foods.

Finally, there is sometimes a direct connection between diet and behavior. Crankiness, irritability, lethargy, uncooperativeness, and many other unproductive behaviors can be influenced by improper diet. Just as emotional problems can influence physical problems, bodily deficiencies can affect how the mind functions and how the child behaves. A practitioner's sensitivity to dietary factors may solve behavioral problems before the child is needlessly taken to a psychologist or psychiatrist.

Dieting

An attempt to limit WEIGHT GAIN by altering either the type or the amount of food eaten.

In children a leveling off of an excessive gain pattern is what is needed, *not* weight loss. If the child is overweight, it is reasonable to limit excesses of sweets and starchy foods. Adequate amounts of protein, fats, and carbohydrates are needed, however, to ensure growth.

As is discussed under DIET, adolescents' self-induced dieting should be strongly discouraged. This is particularly true in teenage girls whose marked weight loss may be connected to ANOREXIA NERVOSA, a serious condition that requires medical and psychiatric care.

Diphtheria

A potentially serious contagious disease caused by *Corynebacterium diphtheriae,* a germ that infects the back of the nose and throat, resulting in a grayish-white membrane that clogs the throat and interferes with breathing.

Formerly a great scourge among infants and young children, diphtheria has been almost eradicated by the introduction of a protective vaccine called DPT. It is unlikely that today's parents will ever encounter the disease. However, in a few instances immunization may have been inadequate. If the child shows a particularly sore throat, difficulty in swallowing, extreme weakness (which can result if the diphtheria toxin is released into the body), and breathing difficulties, be sure to check with the child's doctor. The disease is very serious and may result in severe complications if diphtheria antitoxin is not administered promptly.

Dirty language

See OBSCENE LANGUAGE.

Disability

See LEARNING DISABILITY, PHYSICAL DISABILITY.

Disobedience

The definition depends upon what parents mean by *obedience.* Parents need to discuss this matter between themselves and come to a common understanding of what they mean. That can help to ensure consistency in parental response to behavior that is considered unacceptable. Basically what concerned parents should seek is behavior that meets norms established for the child's age; a gradual socialization through which the child learns the give-and-take of everyday life; and the youngster's growing acceptance of standards of behavior that are acceptable within the home, at school, with other children, and in society at large.

In their zeal to be good parents, many people become overly controlling and too directive. Don't try to mold the child. Let the child make some mistakes and learn from the consequences. Provide general guidance and the means and support so self-respect is acquired. Don't control for the sake of control itself, and do allow the child some time alone, an interval when there are no orders or prohibitions. Having the parent's trust encourages the child to assume responsibility for his or her own behavior.

Before judging the child's behavior as disobedient, remember that from the very beginning, youngsters are striving for independence and self-expression. The way this is expressed often reflects the child's age. Infants tend to express frustration by crying. Toddlers, exploring new ways of getting around and of using newly discovered muscular powers and vocalizations, may throw a TEMPER TANTRUM if they don't get their own way. School-age children may pout, withdraw, or threaten extreme actions such as running away from home. As part of the power struggle between parent and child, conversations may be interrupted, chores left undone, or some behavior embarrassing to the parents be done in public. Adolescence, with its rebelliousness and its demands for real independence and self-assertion, can be a particularly trying time for parents, as it is also for adolescents.

When parents view their child's behavior as continually disobedient, a critical self-appraisal of their parenting techniques may be helpful. Are both parents in agreement about expectations? Is there a consistency of response to unacceptable behavior? Is the child aware of the consequences of misbehavior? Are the methods of discipline fair, and does the punishment fit the crime? If threats of disciplining are made, are they consistently carried out? Is the child being unfairly used to vent parental anxiety or unrest? Is the child experiencing stress that hasn't been explored, perhaps trouble at school or problems with peers? Has *good* behavior been consistently rewarded, and is the child frequently reassured about love and acceptance?

If behavioral difficulties persist after all the factors are inspected and legitimate attempts at change have failed, a discussion with the child's doctor may be in order. Sometimes an objective view can help pinpoint the origin of a particular conflict.

See also: DEPRESSION, AGGRESSIVE BEHAVIOR.

Disorientation

An inability to place oneself properly in terms of person, place, or time.

Sometimes children may experience some degree of disorientation when they wake up in a strange bed, for example, while staying with relatives or in a motel; when they have suddenly awakened from a frightening dream; or when they are ill with a high fever. Usually parental reassurance is all that is needed to bring the child around.

When high fevers are associated with HALLUCINATIONS, the child may become confused and unaware of what is happening. A convulsion is not infrequently followed by some degree of lack of awareness. Disorientation can also result from a child ingesting some toxic or mind-altering substance or from a head injury.

When the disorientation is associated with the acute onset of vomiting, a combative attitude, and the appearance of serious illness, the child may be suffering REYE'S SYNDROME.

Dizziness

The sensation that things seem to be spinning around. Vertigo is a medical term for dizziness. In objective vertigo the surroundings appear to be moving. In subjective vertigo the surroundings seem stationary and the individual feels as though he or she is spinning.

Sometimes as children quickly get up from a sitting or lying position, they may feel lightheaded or giddy. This temporary effect of altered cranial blood pressure is not a true case of vertigo and should cause no parental alarm. Nor would temporary dizziness after spinning in some amusement-park ride qualify as a matter of concern.

Children between the ages of one and four may have episodes of unsteadiness and apparent fright as a result of a middle-ear disorder or infection that interferes with balance, as can also happen with certain drugs taken over a long period of time. Dizziness may also occur after a severe blow to the head that causes a concussion. Vertigo can be confused with SEIZURE DISORDERS, when the attacks do not involve a loss of consciousness. Ménière's syndrome, a middle-ear disorder occasionally seen in older adolescents, is commonly associated with vertigo, vomiting, and tinnitus (ringing in the ears).

Children prone to attacks of dizziness that are not connected with disease states usually grow out of this stage within two or three years.

Double vision

A visual disorder, known technically as diplopia, in which one object is seen as two objects.

The condition may be present from birth, in which case the child usually learns to suppress the vision in one eye. It may be connected to a muscular imbalance that leads to STRABISMUS (a squint). If this situation goes undetected and the child continues to suppress vision in one eye, one-eye blindness may result. If the condition is diagnosed early, it can be treated successfully so that the blindness does not become permanent. If parents notice any such difficulties, they should take the child to an eye specialist at once. On the other hand, children often become quite adept, almost on an unconscious level, at concealing such problems, so a thorough eye examination at around age five is a wise move in any event.

On rare occasion double vision may be one of the first

symptoms of botulism, a severe form of FOOD POISONING caused by *Clostridium botulinum,* an organism that sometimes contaminates improperly preserved food. Prompt medical attention is mandatory, as the toxin (poison) affects the central nervous system and can cause paralysis of the heart and respiratory system.

Down's syndrome

A genetically determined condition in which the child is born with a small and slightly flattened head; distinctive facial characteristics that include slanted eyes (hence the old term "mongolism"), a flat-bridged nose, and a large tongue that tends to protrude; a lack of muscle coordination; short and stubby hands and feet; and varying degrees of mental retardation and slowed physical growth.

Every cell in the body carries chromosomes, microscopic rod-shaped substances that carry hereditary features. Normally every cell in the human male and female carries 23 pairs of chromosomes for a total of 46. In Down's syndrome there is an extra chromosome 21, called trisomy 21, so a Down's syndrome child has 47 chromosomes in each cell. Typically such children are born to women over the age of thirty-five and especially over the age of forty. Yet the disorder can occur in children of younger women, and in approximately one-third of cases studied, the extra chromosome 21 comes from the father.

In addition to the abnormalities listed, some Down's syndrome children have heart defects, and they seem especially prone to develop leukemia. Life expectancy may be shortened, but many people with Down's syndrome survive and enjoy adulthood.

Infants with Down's syndrome rarely cry; they seem quiet and peaceful, show poor muscle tone and little activity, and tend to display little interest in objects and activities that usually fascinate babies. Studies show that children with Down's syndrome who are raised at home usually develop more skills than those who are institutionalized at a very young age, but family circumstances may play a large role in determining if, and when, parents elect to place their child in an appropriate caretaking/educational setting.

Modern advances in prebirth detection may be of help to concerned parents-to-be. Amniocentesis, a process by which a sample of intrauterine fluid is extracted from a pregnant woman, tells doctors whether the fetus has Down's syndrome. This allows parents to consider the possible early termination of a pregnancy, and also to decide whether they should confer with a genetic counselor, who may help them arrive at a decision about not having, or having, other children.

DPT

The initials for a routinely given childhood IMMUNIZATION. The letters stand for the diseases DIPHTHERIA; PERTUSSIS, or whooping cough; and TETANUS. A good degree of protection against those illnesses is provided by the series of injections.

See also: IMMUNIZATION REACTION.

Drooling

Saliva draining outward through the mouth and down over the chin.

Infants who are teething will have increased secretion of saliva; rather than being swallowed, it dribbles outward. Sometimes drooling will continue into the toddler years. Except for wetness of a child's upper clothing, which can be bothersome to fastidious parents, there is no real problem, and the condition generally stops by itself without active treatment.

However, an acutely ill child who has a fever and is experiencing trouble breathing may have a dangerous form of CROUP in which the throat is so sore he or she cannot swallow. This illness can be life threatening, so immediate medical treatment is necessary.

Drowsiness, unusual

The most common reason any child becomes drowsy is obvious—not enough sleep. Sleep patterns vary: some infants will sleep through the night by the time they are only two months old; others will take a night feeding until they are six months or older.

Babies may nap for up to four hours a day, so that they are sleeping about twelve to fourteen hours out of every twenty-four. Toddlers and young children often nap for one to two hours during the day and sleep about eight to ten hours during the night. Growing children and adolescents require at least eight to ten hours of sleep, sometimes more. Parents need to know their own children's patterns if they are going to judge what "unusual drowsiness" is.

Lack of sleep may occur for several reasons: the child goes to bed at an appropriate hour, but sleep does not come until some time afterward; the night may have been one of fitful, irregular sleeping; the child may be worried about something and be afraid to go to sleep (a situation that may be worked out through a reassuring discussion, or may need professional help).

Children who are becoming ill may be unusually tired for a day or two before they develop other symptoms. Certain medications, especially antihistamines, cause drowsiness; so can DEPRESSION or emotional stress. ANEMIA may also produce an undue amount of FATIGABILITY, increasing the need for sleep.

Drug usage

See ADDICTION, WARNING SIGNS OF.

Dysentery

See AMEBIC DYSENTERY, BACILLARY DYSENTERY.

Dyslexia

A significant impairment in the development of reading skills.

There seems to be no single cause of dyslexia. Many factors may be involved. Family histories suggest there may be some genetic component. A previous brain injury or infection could also contribute. The child, more often a boy than a girl, may also have shown slow motor development—that is, poor muscular coordination compared with age peers—and delayed language—that is, not talking as well as age peers. These are signs that parents can recognize while the child is still a preschooler.

It is of utmost importance for parents and teachers to

understand that this impairment has nothing to do with the child's intellectual capacity. Indeed, many dyslexic children are as bright as nondyslexic children. They may, for example, have visual problems in which letters get fused or switched. Sounds may be confused, or the child may have trouble retaining what has gone before other letters or sounds. Both testing and training must be done by experts in the field, not by the average physician or the average teacher. Even after extensive correctional work, dyslexic children often continue to have some difficulties in spelling, reading, and comprehension throughout life. But with proper training, they can be taught to achieve levels that will permit normal achievement in school. Training will also greatly enhance their social acceptance.

E

Earache

Children's brief episodes of earache often reflect nothing more than pressure changes behind the eardrum; they are of no real significance and usually go away without any treatment.

However, ear discomfort may occur because of infections; the presence of a foreign object the child may put in the ear canal, such as insects, pea-size items like stones or parts of toys; direct injury by poking a sharp object into the outer ear canal; or enduring loud blasts. Sometimes pain may spread from the teeth or throat, and, in rare instances, otalgia (ear pain) can be caused by an inflammation of the nerve to the ear.

Frequent or persistent complaints warrant medical evaluation, especially if there is high fever or vomiting. Infants or toddlers who can't yet complain verbally may express ear discomfort by pulling at the ear, rubbing the side of the head, or even banging the head.

Ear drainage

The lining of the outer ear canal produces a continuous supply of earwax, technically called cerumen. Without this wax, itching in the canal would be unbearable.

Earwax makes its way to the outside as a thick, yellow- to brown-colored material that is usually easily removed. When a child has an EAR INFECTION, the eardrum may rupture. Initially a moderate amount of clear, watery drainage appears where earwax usually does. Sometimes blood can be noted. If the condition is not treated, this drainage becomes thick, yellow to green in color, and is foul-smelling. Similar results may occur from poking into the ear canal, from the presence of a foreign body lodged in the outer canal, or from a HEAD INJURY. Prompt medical attention is a must, especially for the latter.

Ear infection

Any infection affecting the outer, middle, or inner portion of the ear.

Some children seem unusually prone to ear infections. Because the three separate portions of the human ear may show different kinds of infections and their related symptoms, parents need to know a little bit about these anatomical areas. You can see the outermost portion of the outer ear canal. It is a tubelike structure that leads inward to a thin membrane called the eardrum. Sound waves pass from here into the middle ear, where small bones work to further transmit sound and where the eustachian tube helps equalize air pressure. In the inner ear lie structures that convert sound waves into nerve impulses (to be transferred to the brain for processing) and help maintain a person's sense of equilibrium or balance.

Otitis externa (outer ear infection) often occurs when a child has been playing in swimming water that carries bacteria or funguses. The lining of the canal swells and drains and becomes quite painful. Fever or nasal congestion is rarely present, but the child will complain vigorously if the ear is pressed or the earlobe is tugged. Treatment consists of special drops prescribed by a physician, which often can also be used just before and just after swimming, to help prevent recurrences. If the canal is swollen shut, some temporary loss of hearing will be evident, but outer canal infections do not affect hearing on a permanent basis. Occasionally a "spillover" of infected material will spread infection from the middle ear; in this case, too, treatment will probably be of eardrops prescribed for the external component of the infection.

Otitis media (middle ear infection) is more frequent; few children and adolescents seem to escape at least one bout. Blockage of the eustachian tube is a common cause. Usually a middle ear infection is preceded by signs of a common cold with nasal congestion and cough. Approximately 60 percent of the time a fever will be present, with temperatures of over 101°F (38.3°C). A doctor will generally prescribe an antibiotic, not so much for the ear problem itself (which may be minimal and may clear up) but to avoid a more serious infection such as MASTOIDITIS or MENINGITIS.

Once the acute symptoms of a middle ear infection have

cleared, the child should be rechecked to make sure there is no fluid left in the cavity of the middle ear, which could thicken and interfere with the workings of the tiny bones there or cause a rupture of the eardrum because of increased pressure.

Otitis interna or labyrinthitis (inner ear infection) is not common during childhood. On occasion it may occur when infection spreads inward from the middle ear or downward from the meninges (the three membranes that cover the brain). Sometimes an inner ear infection may be associated with influenza. Common signs are dizziness (vertigo), tinnitus (ringing in the ear), and partial or total loss of hearing in the affected ear. Symptoms are frequently worse when the child makes a sudden movement of the head or sits up suddenly. Treatment depends on the severity of the infection and, of course, on whether it has spread from such a delicate site as the brain. Usually antibiotics and bed rest will clear up an inner ear infection.

Parents should keep in mind that children's ear problems tend to recur. If you have eardrops previously prescribed for the same child within the past year, you may use them; but be sure to call the child's doctor if the problem persists. *Never* use an adult's prescription (such as an antibiotic) or another child's medication to treat a child who may have an ear infection. Even when the discomfort eases, the child should probably be examined by a doctor to make sure that the infection is controlled and that there is no fluid behind the ear drum. Because of children's susceptibility to upper respiratory infections, recurrences of ear problems can be expected. Parents should not be alarmed by these recurrences as long as each episode is promptly and properly treated.

Ear, noises in

See TINNITUS.

Eczema

A skin rash characterized by redness, itching, scaling, and crusting; in some cases, blistering may occur.

In children, eczema is usually related to an ALLERGY, and the youngster is apt to suffer other allergic reactions, such as asthma.

In infants, the condition usually occurs between about six months and one year, with reddish colored, crusty raised marks on the cheeks. Sometimes a parent will notice cracks behind the child's ears. Often lesions will appear on the arms and legs, especially in the depressions in front of the elbows and behind the knees. Another form of the disorder generally occurs in children over the age of one. The lesions are raised and roundish, often filled with fluid, and intensely itchy.

The most serious form of eczema, called generalized eczema, is most often encountered in children over four years old. Almost the entire body is covered with running, crusty, itchy skin eruptions.

The child's doctor may prescribe cortisone and a medicated lotion, and possibly a special diet that restricts milk intake. Parents can provide some relief from the itching by not bathing the child so often and by using cornstarch or bath oils in the bath water as a means of decreasing skin dryness. It is wise to follow commonsense hygienic measures in efforts to avoid secondary bacterial infections of skin that is already ravaged by eczema.

Medical treatment is essential, not only for general supervision of treatment, which may include antihistamines and the use of corticosteroid compounds, but also for emotional counseling. Children may subconsciously use their eczema to exercise undue control over the family; also, stress tends to worsen the disease. This could lead to a vicious cycle of emotional instability for parents and the family in general.

Edema

A swelling of body tissue, which can be local or general.

Sometimes the child develops localized swelling as a result of some injury. Damage to the walls of small blood vessels may permit seepage of fluid into tissue spaces. Similar edema may be caused by allergic irritations and infections.

More generalized or widespread edema may occur when a child has serious kidney disease or heart disease. Any edema that seems unduly extensive or cannot be explained by some known injury or other irritant should certainly alert the parents to seek prompt medical attention for their child.

Emotional withdrawal

A form of behavior in which children or adolescents stop engaging in activities or relationships that previously seemed quite meaningful to them.

Emotional withdrawal may be a prominent feature of a childhood DEPRESSION, and if a clear pattern emerges of shunning friends and avoiding family and other social interactions, parents may want to seek professional help. Sometimes short-term family therapy is effective.

On the other hand, changing interests are a normal part of growing up. A youngster who last year seemed to do nothing but climb trees may suddenly opt for the studious and rather solitary activity of stamp collecting. Preadolescents and adolescents may go through painful periods of shyness as they try to cope with a new body image and newly awakened interests. Often children welcome discussions with their parents if they are approached in a serious, sympathetic, and nonteasing manner. If the areas of concern can't be defined or if the withdrawal seems unduly severe and prolonged, check with the child's doctor. Perhaps counseling is in order, or perhaps there is some physical cause for the child's subdued state.

Encephalitis

An inflammation of the brain. It is a fairly broad diagnostic term that also covers certain kinds of inflammations that are of noninfectious origins, for example, as a complication of other diseases, disorders, or diagnostic procedures. However, most commonly encephalitis is caused by a viral infection. The infection may be spread by virus-carrying insects or animals with rabies, or it may be a complication of viral diseases such as measles, chickenpox, influenza, mumps, and infectious mononucleosis. Parents should be reassured that rarely do the common childhood illnesses like measles lead to encephalitis, but it is a possibility.

Aside from the symptom of stiff neck, which could also indicate MENINGITIS, with which the disease can be confused until appropriate diagnostic tests are performed, the first evidence of the disease is not very specific. Children may show fever, which may induce disordered thinking or even hallucinations; intensely severe headache; protracted, almost unrelenting vomiting; and lethargy that may progress to coma. Convulsions, temper outbursts, bizarre movements, hyperactivity, and loss of bowel and bladder control may occur.

Treatment is basically aimed at maintaining life and overcoming impaired functioning of vital organ systems such as the lungs and heart. If a BACTERIAL INFECTION is suspected, or at least until it is firmly excluded as a cause, physicians usually inject antibiotics as a precaution.

Encephalitis is extremely serious. It demands prompt medical attention. Therefore, even if the disease's first signs and symptoms seem rather unspecific, parents should immediately seek medical help when children show the slightest evidence of possible encephalitis.

Compare MENINGITIS.

Endocarditis

An inflammation of the membrane called the endocardium, which lines the heart and its valves.

It usually occurs as a result of bacteria trapped around the heart valves. Before the advent of antibiotics, endocarditis was frequently one of the dangerous aftermaths of RHEUMATIC FEVER. Modern treatment consists of a prolonged course of antibiotics; bed rest is no longer considered necessary. Those children who have structural heart disease (valve or septal defects) should be given preventive antibiotic therapy before dental work or before certain types of surgery are performed so that endocarditis is avoided.

Enteritis

See GASTROENTERITIS, REGIONAL ENTERITIS.

Enuresis

See BEDWETTING.

Epiglottitis

See CROUP.

Epilepsy

See SEIZURE DISORDERS.

Epistaxis

See NOSEBLEED.

Eye drainage

Some infants are born with a blocked tear duct, which causes a clear, watery discharge from the eye because the tears can't drain properly. When the tears dry they form a yellow crusting on the lids and in the corners of the eye. The white of the eye, however, does not looked inflamed or reddened. Gentle cleansing with water is all that is needed.

Several common diseases of childhood cause temporary tearing. Sometimes blockage of the tear duct, as mentioned, causes infants to have an increased risk of developing an eye infection. When this happens the discharge is continuous and puslike, and the white of the eye is reddened. Treatment includes antibiotic eyedrops, and the doctor may instruct parents how to gently massage along the corner of the baby's eye and down along the side of the nose to encourage drainage. If the condition does not clear up, an ophthalmologist (eye specialist) may need to probe the duct, an operation that is performed under general anesthesia. This probing is usually not done before the child is one year old.

Children may develop various eye infections that cause thick, yellow drainage and an inflamed, reddish-colored eyeball. Eye drainage associated with itching may signal the presence of allergies. Proper treatment depends on the doctor's specific diagnosis.

Eye, foreign body in

Flecks of foreign material, such as dirt or dust, are usually washed away by an immediate flow of tears. If this doesn't work, and gentle flooding with water or a sterile solution fails to dislodge the material, removal should probably be undertaken only by a doctor, nurse, or other practitioner who is trained to do this.

Larger objects, or ones that strike the eye with force, may scratch the cornea (the transparent covering in front of the eyeball) or the conjunctiva (the membrane that lines the eyelid and covers the white of the eye). The child is usually in extreme discomfort; tearing is common, the eye looks quite red. Because tiny scratches in these delicate linings may provide an entry for harmful microorganisms, the child should be examined by a doctor. A special staining technique permits accurate location of the injury, and appropriate medications can be prescribed.

Any injury that penetrates into the eyeball is very serious. Never attempt to remove the object. Simply cover the eye with a cool wet cloth and rush the child to a doctor or the nearest emergency medical facility.

Eye infection

Both viruses and bacteria can cause eye infection. At first the eye may appear red, with a clear, watery drainage. Itchiness usually causes the child to rub the eye, which aggravates the symptoms. As the infection becomes worse, the drainage becomes thickened and turns yellow-green.

When the itching subsides, the child shows marked discomfort when exposed to a strong light and he or she complains, verbally or by crying, of considerable pain.

Since the eye is such a sensitive and important organ, professional evaluation and treatment are necessary. Prescription antibiotic drops are usually given.

Eye itching

An eye irritation that causes prolonged itching may occur because of an allergy or an eye infection. In either case the child should be seen by a physician.

Occasionally smoke or other airborne substances cause the eyes to itch or burn. Once the child is removed from this situation, the eyes soon stop itching.

Eye, lazy

See STRABISMUS.

Eyelid swelling

Swelling of both upper and lower eyelids is a common finding in EYE INFECTIONS. In newborn babies, lid swelling may be a sign of spreading infection requiring prompt medical attention, especially if the swelling extends onto the face or forehead.

An allergy can cause the lids to swell, often rapidly. Small, localized swellings of the lids may be found when a STYE, a CYST, or an insect bite is present.

Eyelid swelling also occurs in diseases that cause retention of fluids, such as kidney disorders. When this is the case, other symptoms are present and most likely the child is already under medical supervision.

Eye pain

While eye discomfort commonly occurs with fatigue, children who *recurrently* complain of eye discomfort should be checked by a physician.

Chronic eyestrain from poor vision may cause pain. Eye pain may also be associated with several disorders, including migraine HEADACHES, SINUSITIS, and the very serious infection ENCEPHALITIS.

Eye redness

Small blood vessels abound in the eye, and they are responsible for the reddened or bloodshot appearance of irritated eyes. Eyestrain from poor vision and generalized fatigue from overexertion or lack of sleep may cause red eyes. Nonprescription eyedrops or ointments may offer some relief, but if the redness persists or recurs, or other symptoms are present, a doctor's evaluation is advisable.

Bloodshot eyes may occur when an EYE INFECTION or ALLERGY is present.

See also: CONJUNCTIVITIS.

F

Facial pain

In addition to obvious injuries or infections, other medical conditions may give rise to facial pain.

Children with SINUSITIS frequently complain of facial discomfort, and sometimes the swelling over the sinus is noticeable. Sometimes pain from a toothache or dental abscess is felt as facial pain. Migraine headaches are sometimes associated with pain felt around or behind one of the eyes.

More rarely, tumors or cysts of the facial bones cause some degree of pain. In even rarer circumstances an inflammation of a cranial nerve that registers sensation in the face causes severe facial pain.

When the child's complaint of facial pain cannot be easily explained, parents should seek medical advice.

Facial swelling

The commonest cause of facial swelling is an insect bite. Often children don't recall being bitten (and may have been unaware when they were), or the bite may go unnoticed once swelling has occurred, especially if it's around the eyes.

Application of cool, wet compresses will offer some relief, and a doctor or pharmacist may be able to suggest something to ease the pain such swelling usually causes.

Other causes of facial swelling may involve mumps, sinusitis, swollen glands, or dental conditions. More serious medical conditions such as cysts and tumors or acute kidney inflammations may cause facial swelling. When an infant or young child rapidly develops any reddened facial swelling and a fever (102°F or 39°C), one might suspect a serious bacterial infection, which demands intravenously administered antibiotics on an urgent basis.

Fainting

A temporary loss of consciousness and muscle control, technically known as syncope.

A simple fainting spell is not uncommon in childhood. It occurs because of a rapid drop in blood pressure in vessels supplying the brain and heart. It can, for example, be brought about by too quickly rising to an upright position. But children often faint when they are suddenly frightened, embarrassed, or in pain. Some children briefly lose consciousness over the simple removal of a splinter in the finger. Others, particularly older children or adolescents, may faint in response to some emotional strain that is experienced as overwhelming, such as having to give a speech or perform at a concert, or feeling clumsy when encountering someone who awes them.

The child may at first feel lightheaded and dizzy, and the skin becomes clammy. Occasionally there may be a brief twitching of muscles in the arms and face. Usually vision grows dim and fuzzy until the child simply blacks out and collapses, or gradually sinks to the floor or ground.

When the child complains of feeling faint, tilting the head downward at a 45-degree angle often helps prevent a total faint. Otherwise, simply help the child lie down if he or she has not already collapsed. Usually these attacks are brief and leave no ill effects afterward. Parents may wish to discuss their children's fainting spell(s) with a doctor, just in case some other condition such as abnormal heart rhythms or some SEIZURE DISORDERS may be present.

Fallen arches

See FLAT FEET.

Falling

Young children's behavior tends to be impulsive; they don't think before acting. As part of this pattern, children run or climb before they look at what might be in their way. Frequent falls and bruises are the rule rather than the exception.

It is not possible for parents to protect youngsters from their own tangled feet. Nor should this necessarily be attempted; children need to test newly discovered muscular coordination. Falls and scraped legs are a normal part of young children's everyday life.

Parents need, however, to be alert to signs of staggering

or undue unsteadiness that might indicate an inflammation of the inner ear, where balance mechanisms are located. Other signs such as tremors, muscle weakness, and a wobbly gait might suggest a neurological disorder, as might the child's sudden fall to one side or the other even though he or she is not particularly active at the moment. These situations call for a doctor's diagnosis and treatment.

Farsightedness

A visual disorder, technically known as hyperopia or hypermetropia, that occurs when the eyeball is too short from front to back. As a result of this abnormality, light is focused slightly behind the retina and the child sees blurred images of objects that are close to the eye. Vision for faraway objects is not affected, so the condition is called farsightedness.

Most babies are somewhat farsighted at birth. As the eye grows during normal development, it usually allows the lens to focus images directly on the retina. Occasionally the shape of the eyeball continues to remain too short from front to back. For a time the lens can adjust by changing its shape so that rays of light are focused where they should be. But in order to accomplish this, the eye's ciliary muscles are under tension for long periods of time, which can cause eyestrain and headaches until the condition is corrected.

Parents should be sure their preschooler's eyes are examined, especially if signs of strain are evident. In less severe forms of farsightedness, corrective lenses may have to be worn only when the child is reading or doing other close work.

Compare NEARSIGHTEDNESS.

Fatal illness

See TERMINAL ILLNESS.

Fatigability

Along with the emotional mood swings seen in adolescence, there is an associated shift in energy levels. Many teenagers seem to require great amounts of sleep and may act as though they're always tired. Rapid growth, changes in metabolism, and the energy expended on emotional development are draining.

All children, including toddlers and youngsters, may become fatigued simply by too much physical exertion and insufficient rest or sleep. However, stress may add to children's fatigability. If gentle discussion cannot uncover family, peer, or school difficulties that may be stressful, some professional counseling may help. Parents should also keep in mind that unusual fatigability may indicate the subtle presence of some medical condition; therefore, a physical checkup might be in order.

See also: ANEMIA; DEPRESSION; DROWSINESS, UNUSUAL.

Fears

Mental-health professionals often make a distinction between fear and anxiety. Fear is generally characterized as a reasonable reaction to something real that is generally looked upon as threatening or frightening. One could call a phobia *unreasonable* fear because it is highly exaggerated over what most people, including children, commonly experience. Anxiety is often tied to more vague fears that do not seem to be related to things that are readily seen, felt, or understood.

For most parents the distinction may be more confusing than helpful. This is certainly true for the children themselves. Perhaps many fears are symbolic in origin and represent other anxieties, for example, dreading parental punishment or loss of parental love. Sometimes children become somewhat preoccupied with such concerns and behave anxiously in an overall way; that is, they may become jumpy, withdrawn, tearful, overexcited, hard to get along with. If this becomes a marked problem, parents may want to discuss the matter with the child's doctor, who can help provide some guidance or perhaps make a referral for counseling.

In the vast majority of cases, the child's fears dissipate with calm parental reassurance and the child's own emotional growth as he or she gains more confidence.

Children should never be forcefully made to experience something they fear just to prove nothing will happen. For example, making a screaming child sit in a swing while you push it or shutting off the lights when the youngster is afraid of the dark only reinforces the fear. Children are apt to become even more fearful because parents have exposed them to a danger they consider very real, even if it's not. If the child is afraid of the dark, allowing a night light in his or her room, coupled with gentle reminders that ghosts and monsters do not exist, is far more effective.

Obviously, everyone has fears. It is only when they seem to interfere with the child's functional level that any attention should be directed at correction. A direct behavioral approach seems to work better than endless discussions of the fear. In fact, this could backfire by turning the fear into an attention-seeking device.

Fecal soiling

Children who begin to have accidents with bowel movements long after they are toilet trained may be doing so because they are trying to avoid having a bowel movement at all.

This condition is seen more frequently in boys than in girls. The child may fight the urge to go to the bathroom to avoid interrupting play or other activities. Resistance during school hours may indicate the child is uncomfortable in a strange bathroom or is embarrassed by the need to go to the bathroom at all. In some cases either a series of diarrheal episodes or having previously had a large and painful bowel movement may cause the child to be fearful that it will hurt again. Some authorities consider fecal soiling a sign of severe psychological disturbance, but, unless it is accompanied by other emotional symptoms, the situation does not require any special counseling. Whatever the cause, and often it simply cannot be determined, the child begins to resist going to the bathroom.

An early sign is cramping abdominal pain, which occurs because the child is holding back and fighting the urge to go. When successful, a day or two might pass without a bowel movement. When the child does go, the stool is large and likely to cause discomfort in passing.

Gradually the period between bowel movements lengthens. Large amounts of stool are present in the lower intestine, so that underclothing may be soiled several times a day as fluid or small amounts of formed fecal material leak around the impacted stool. If this pattern persists longer than six to twelve months, the intestinal wall loses some of its normal tone because it is stretched by the frequent collection of waste matter. At this point a physical cause for constipation and infrequent stooling exists.

What is necessary is to reestablish a normal bowel pattern and keep the bowel as free as possible from large collections of stool. This retraining should begin as soon as parents become aware of the problem, at which point they should consult the child's doctor. The physician may recommend enemas, stool softeners, or suppositories for rectal stimulation. This should be scheduled for a convenient time each day, preferably at the same time each day. Laxatives should *not* be used. As the child becomes accustomed to regular bowel movements and understands that he will have to go in spite of any holding, he gradually relearns normal toilet habits. Soiling is reduced because there is no excess buildup of stool, so corresponding embarrassment over accidents dissipates.

See also: BOWEL MOVEMENT.

Feeding pattern changes

The frequency and amount of feedings during infancy depend mostly on the baby's growth requirements. For the first few weeks an infant will want to eat small amounts frequently. If too much is offered and taken, it will be graciously returned on the burping cloth on your shoulder.

After about six weeks, a feeding in the middle of the night is really not necessary. Substituting water will help. It may take a few days, but most babies will "decide" it's really not worth getting up at two o'clock in the morning for a couple of ounces of water.

Solid foods need not be introduced until an infant is about four months old, when, as a rule, the swallowing mechanisms and digestive systems are better prepared to accept them. As more solids are introduced, the amount of milk needed diminishes. Since vegetables, fruits, and meats have fewer calories per ounce than milk, excessive weight gain is avoided. By the age of six or seven months the infant should be on a schedule that will approach what childhood patterns will be: a carbohydrate source for breakfast: cereal and fruit; something filling but not fattening for lunch: vegetable and perhaps fruit; and a protein source for dinner: meat, vegetable.

Amounts and consistency will depend on what the baby can handle without choking or gagging. Finger foods, more to be played with than eaten, help develop coordination and allow the baby to begin to learn self-feeding.

When an infant reaches one year of age and weighs about twenty pounds, a rather dramatic decrease in appetite occurs. This often concerns parents, but it needn't. The change merely means that the child has reached a predictable and normal slowdown in growth rate.

Compare APPETITE CHANGES.

Feet

See FLAT FEET, TOEING-IN, TOEING-OUT.

Fever

A rise in body temperature above 100°F (37.8°C) when the measurement is taken rectally. If the child's temperature cannot be taken rectally, you can gain some approximation by taking it orally or in the armpit (axillary region). Ranges for normal body temperature are:

Rectal	98°–100°F	36.6°–37.8°C
Oral	97°–99°F	36.1°–37.1°C
Axillary	96°–98°F	35.6°–36.6°C

Keep the thermometer in place at least three minutes.

Accuracy of temperature may vary for many reasons other than body site, measuring technique, or presence of illness. Temperature of the surrounding air can cause some variation in body temperature. Vigorous play or environmental heat may cause readings of up to 100.5°F (38.1°C). Body temperature tends to swing from one time of day to another. This change, caused by varying secretion of cortisone by the adrenal glands, may cause lower readings in the morning and higher readings later in the day. If a child has been drinking cold liquids immediately before an oral temperature is taken, the reading will be artificially lowered.

A fever serves two purposes: alerting one to the possibility of disease and fighting, in a natural way, that disease or illness. In other words, vigorous attempts at fever reduction may sometimes delay accurate diagnosis and the body's own attempt to rid itself of sickness.

Therefore, except in young infants in the first few months of life, temperatures up to 102°F (38.9°C) need not be treated. Actually it is only in rare circumstances that a fever produces ill effects on the body. Temperatures below 107°F (41.5°C) do not cause brain damage; some infants and children have suffered no permanent injury as the result of short-term temperatures even up to 109°F (42.8°C). Parents often have an unreasonable fear that if children's fevers get too high, the youngsters will suffer a convulsion (see FEVER CONVULSION). As a matter of fact, if a seizure does occur, it often happens as the fever is just beginning its climb upward, not when it peaks. There is also a great deal of individual variation in sensitivity to temperature changes. Above all, since fever convulsions are not particularly dangerous, a concentrated attempt at keeping the child's temperature down serves little purpose.

Other factors, such as age and the presence of other signs or symptoms, are more important. For example, if a rectal temperature higher than 100°F (37.8°C) or lower than 97.5°F (36.6°C) occurs in an infant six weeks old or younger, that baby should be immediately taken for a medical examination. In very young babies serious infections may be heralded by sudden fever or an abnormally low temperature.

The presence of signs and symptoms other than fever must be considered. For example, a temperature of only 102°F (39°C) in the child who has a stiff neck and is vomiting is far, far more serious than one of 104°F (40°C) in an infant who looks well and is acting fairly well. In the first instance the child may have MENINGITIS; in the second ROSEOLA, a rather harmless illness.

How does the child look and act as the temperature comes down? If activity and appearance improve, the illness is probably not urgent. But when children look as ill with 100.5°F (38°C) as they did at 103°F (39.5°C), parents should call a doctor at once.

What happens when the temperature increases rapidly? Parents frequently express concern about a temperature that suddenly shot up to 105°F. Some fevers do progress rapidly, but no child's temperature is 98.6°F one minute and 105°F the next. It's simply that the parent didn't know about it and wasn't measuring it when it was 101°, 102°, 103°, 104°, then 105°F.

When the doctor agrees that it's best to try to bring the fever down, several things can be done. Aspirin or acetaminophen compounds can be administered, but parents should be sure to follow label directions very carefully. Aspirin should not be used if the child has an influenzalike illness or chickenpox because of a possible link to a serious complication called REYE'S SYNDROME.

If the child's temperature is under 105°F, external cooling, such as by sponging, may not be necessary. However, it often offers the child some comfort. Immersing a feverish child in cool water accomplishes little; nor does wrapping him or her in cold wet towels. The best method involves placing the naked child on a large towel. Using a washcloth or your hands, gently apply tepid water all over the body. Wait a few minutes for some drying to occur, then repeat the process. Check the child's temperature every twenty minutes. Don't be concerned if it hasn't come down; it may even go up a bit more. Sometimes it can be brought down in twenty minutes; sometimes it takes an hour.

Never use alcohol, alone or in water, for sponging. It may be absorbed into the body and cause toxic (poisoning) effects.

Parents can best be prepared to deal with children's fevers if they follow a plan. Early in the infant's life, discuss with the baby's doctor how he or she prefers to manage fevers, and when and under what circumstances the child's doctor should be called. Keep a fever-reducing medicine at home, in dosage forms appropriate for the youngster and approved by the doctor.

These steps should prepare you for most fever circumstances. However, when other symptoms are present along with the fever, or whenever a fever has persisted for more than twenty-four hours, call the child's doctor to discuss the condition.

See also: BODY TEMPERATURE.
Compare HYPOTHERMIA.

Fever blister

See COLD SORE, HERPES SIMPLEX.

Fever convulsion

Usually a brief episode of generalized seizure (involuntary muscle movements) brought on by fever and associated with a loss of consciousness. Jerking movements of the extremities and trunk are common and may be quite vigorous.

Fever convulsions occur in some 3 percent to 5 percent of otherwise healthy children, more often in boys than in girls. Although the convulsions may be seen as late as ages six to eight, they usually occur between six months and two or three years of age, with a peak at around eighteen months. Parents should be reassured that fever convulsions are not usually significant and appear to be something most children outgrow. They occur most commonly when there is a rapid and sudden temperature rise.

Although there is generally no harm done by the seizure itself, the child should certainly be protected. If vomiting occurs, the parent should turn the child's head to one side and keep the airway clear. Be certain that breathing continues after the convulsion. The child should then be wrapped warmly and taken immediately to an emergency medical facility. After a first such seizure, a spinal tap may be taken if doctors suspect meningitis, a disorder that also causes generalized convulsions.

Long-term management will depend on the age of the child, the number of times seizures have occurred, family history of fever seizures, and certain diagnostic tests such as the electroencephalogram (EEG), which measures brain waves.

Fidgeting

Frequent and sometimes almost ritualistic movements of an extremity or of the body in general. Often a signal of some ATTENTION DEFICIT DISORDERS, fidgeting is a part of other symptoms and signs of increased activity.

See also: RESTLESS BEHAVIOR.

Fifth disease

The disease, known medically as erythema infectiosum, is often called fifth disease because it is the fifth of other illnesses that produce somewhat similar rashes. The other four illnesses are rubella, measles, scarlet fever, and a rare and mild form of scarlet fever called Filatov-Dukes disease.

Fifth disease is a mild viral infection of childhood that features a sudden and typical face rash with a "slapped cheek" appearance. The rash, which may also appear on the trunk and limbs, eventually fades into a pink, mottled, lacelike pattern, and there is usually little or no fever. After an incubation period of approximately one week, the illness may last up to ten days, with the rash persisting or recurring off and on for another two or three weeks.

Complications are rare and no treatment is necessary. Therefore a child with fifth disease need not be isolated or kept from attending school.

Fighting

See AGGRESSIVE BEHAVIOR.

Fingernails

See NAILS.

Fire setting

At one time or another most children are fascinated by matches and fire.

With proper parental guidance, all children learn the risks such play involves. So it is generally only when the interest is preoccupying and children actually set dangerous fires that professional help is necessary. Fire setting is most likely accompanied by other signs of antisocial behavior, such as stealing, lying, or displaying undue aggression toward others.

Flat feet

It is normal for babies and small youngsters to have flat feet. The connective tissues in their feet are very soft and pliable. When these young children stand, it seems as though the arch flattens completely. However, when they sit, you can see a very definite curve to the bottom of the foot. As growth continues, the arch will strengthen regardless of whether shoes are worn. Parents should also know that the arch is variable from one child to another. Only about 15 percent of children have no arch at all, a condition generally called fallen arches.

Except for a type of flat foot caused by a tight heel cord, in which stretching exercises may help, there is usually no treatment prescribed. Sometimes special shoes may provide more comfort, but the correction exists only when the shoes are worn. Pads sometimes used to build up an arch may produce discomfort where there wasn't any.

Flu

See INFLUENZA.

Fontanel

Often referred to as the soft spot, the fontanel is that area parents are aware of near the front of the baby's skull. It is an area covered with strong fibrous tissue that has not yet turned to bone. There is a wide variation in the time it takes for this tissue to become bony, but this is usually accomplished by the time a baby is eighteen months old.

This juncture point is really quite strong, and parents need not be unduly concerned about hurting the infant's head.

Food poisoning

An acute illness caused by eating food that has been contaminated with pathogenic (disease-causing) bacteria or food that contains natural poisons, such as eating poisonous toadstools mistaken for harmless mushrooms.

The commonest form of food poisoning is caused by eating food contaminated by the staphylococcal germ. These bacteria multiply in food that has been left in opened and unrefrigerated cans, or in food that has been improperly canned or preserved, or in meats and other foods left too long in warmth or heat (an environment that favors rapid growth of bacteria).

The incubation period—the time from eating contaminated food to the onset of the first symptoms of the disease—is usually only a matter of a few hours. Staphylococcal food poisoning causes GASTROENTERITIS (inflammation of the lining of the stomach and intestines), usually causing diarrhea and vomiting and sometimes draining the body of enough fluids and essential mineral salts to create DEHYDRATION, a condition particularly harmful to infants.

Fluids can usually be replaced by drinking solutions such as Pedialyte or Lytren. The liquid should be cool and should be sipped very slowly, using a teaspoon if necessary, to prevent the recurrence of vomiting.

Another cause of food poisoning is contamination with a bacteria known as *salmonella.* Some pets, especially turtles, may be transmitters of the disease. Salmonellosis usually is not severe and clears within a matter of days. Only if DEHYDRATION or a very ill appearance is present is there a need for antibiotic or intravenous therapy.

Sometimes the illnesses last only one or two days and may be so mild that medical treatment is not required. But the doctor should certainly be notified when children are first suspected of experiencing symptoms of food poisoning. Botulism, a much more serious form of food poisoning, may have to be considered. If possible, the doctor should be given a sample of the food that's suspected of having caused the illness.

Forgetful behavior

A form of behavior in which the child seemingly ignores the directions of parents or other authority figures. When confronted, the youngster simply says, "I forgot."

Most children at one time or another forget to bring homework from school, clean their room, take out the garbage, and so on. Loud reprimands accomplish little. Remarking about the oversight and perhaps restricting a certain privilege may help children become aware that their behavior has certain consequences.

Despite the fact that some authorities would argue that forgetfulness represents a passive form of aggression, simply not doing what is told rather than fighting or arguing, thereby risking loss of parental love, few children need professional help unless forgetfulness is accompanied by other signs, such as falling performance in school, poor interpersonal relationships, or vague physical symptoms. Also parents should remember that children are active both physically and emotionally. In their rapid pace of emotional growth, children may indeed really forget to do something that was asked of them. An occasional slip ought to go unpunished, although not unnoticed.

Fracture

A break in the normal structure of a bone or a tooth, usually the result of an injury. Pain at the site of injury is a predominant symptom. Parents may also note swelling and discoloration of the overlying tissues. At times a loss of contour will be noticeable. Children may also experience numbness in an extremity, a pale demeanor, and, especially in infants and toddlers, fussiness and irritability. Any rapid discoloration farther out in the extremity from the site of injury may mean damage to a major blood vessel; emergency surgery may be necessary.

Occasionally fractures—especially of the collarbone—may occur at delivery, and attending physicians will treat it at that time. Collarbone fractures are also not uncommon in infants or toddlers, who may simply stop using the arm on the affected side and/or cry when the arm is moved. Special bandages can be applied to lessen the discomfort as healing takes place.

At times, seemingly minor acts such as jumping off a chair are sufficient to break a bone in the lower leg. And the falls common to childhood result fairly often in broken arms.

When a fracture is suspected, restrict movement of the affected part and take the child to an emergency room or a physician's office. The doctor will generally use X ray to confirm the nature of the fracture, then realign the bone, then immobilize the affected part, usually in a cast. Parents should be sure they receive thorough instructions about cast care, especially if the child is too young to carry any of the responsibility.

Freckles

Small red- to brown-colored spots on the skin, usually most prevalent in areas most exposed to sunlight like the face, neck, and arms. They occur because of increased production of a pigment and they tend to run in families, being most common in children who have red or reddish hair.

There is no medical significance to freckles. Avoiding frequent or heavy exposure to sunlight makes them less obvious, and certain cosmetics are available to conceal them if appearance becomes a concern.

Frostbite

Damage to the skin caused by exposure to extreme cold. Fingers, toes, ears, and the nose are most commonly stricken. Immediate treatment consists of simply allowing the affected areas to rewarm slowly. Do *not* immerse in hot water, rub with snow or attempt massage. Do *not,* as used to be recommended, immerse in cold water, either.

If sensation and normal coloring do not return within a short time, consult the child's doctor at once. Permanent damage or even gangrene (localized death of the affected tissues) can result if medical treatment is delayed.

Frustration

When needs or desires—even unrealistic ones—are not met, one feels a sense of anger and frustration. Part of a child's maturing concerns learning to live with frustration.

In their impulsivity, infants and very young children seem to demand immediate gratification; they feel frustrated when their wants are thwarted. Parents should not strive to protect their children from all frustration. Youngsters constantly set up circumstances that test their newly discovered control of themselves and the environment. When they learn that no great ill befalls them if everything does not go exactly their way, they develop tolerance for disappointing events. They learn to deal with unsatisfied goals.

Learning adjustment and compromise is not easy. Children may react to seemingly trivial setbacks with anger, a crying spell, or refusal to continue an activity. Only if this pattern continues and seems to occur regularly might a parent consider seeking some professional help. A short ATTENTION SPAN, excess motor activity, ATTENTION DEFICIT DISORDERS and DEPRESSION may signal a disturbance beyond a young child's normal attempts at learning to deal effectively with frustration. As always, age is an important factor. A slip of a pencil may result in a crumpled drawing for a three-year-old. A slightly crooked wing may end up in a crushed airplane model for a six-year-old. If the child engaging in this intolerant behavior is, for example, eight or ten, then a professional counsultation is in order.

Funerals

Before the age of seven or eight, the average child does not have much understanding of the finality of death. Even until age ten, children may be rather confused by the event.

Unless a youngster is unusually mature, viewing a body in a funeral home and witnessing all the grief surrounding a funeral may be extremely anxiety provoking. Children under age five or six should, if possible, be left at home if their parents must attend a funeral. Children who are seven or older may attend if they've been properly prepared. After age ten children are less apt to have an adverse reaction, but even then some preparatory conversation is helpful.

Those who propose that even a very young child should attend funerals or viewings maintain that children need to learn to deal with loss and grieving. This may be true, but it is probably wiser to let them learn these things when they are older. The anxiety caused is likely to be far greater than any benefits. If someone close to the parents dies, children will learn something of grief by sharing their reactions.

Death should never be explained as sleep. Some children may try to avoid sleeping, for fear they might die. In families who believe in a life hereafter, children can be told that the person who has died is now enjoying a different kind of existence in another place. If the concept of an afterlife is not part of the family's beliefs, the child can be told that the one who has died can no longer be part of their everyday lives, but that the survivors can take pleasure in remembering all the past experiences they have shared with the deceased.

If it is the child's own parent or sibling who has died, many other factors come into play; decisions must be individualized.

When there is really no way to avoid a child's attendance at a viewing or a funeral, or the family (and, on occasion, the child) feel strongly that participation is desirable, it is a good idea to see that the child is accompanied by someone who is not deeply involved in the grieving and who can offer some objective explanations of what is happening.

See also: DEATH.

Fungus infection

The fungus family includes a wide variety of primitive plant life —molds, mushrooms, toadstools, yeasts, mildew and many other simple microorganisms. Not all of them are harmful to the body, and only a relative few are capable of infecting the skin.

Tinea (ringworm) has nothing to do with worms; it is merely the name of a group of parasitic fungi that may infect the hands, nails, scalp, feet (ATHLETE'S FEET) and groin (JOCK ITCH). Itching and the redness of inflammation are the most common first signs. Early treatment consists of applying medicated preparations, frequent and careful washing of the affected area and at least daily changes of socks or underwear. However, fungi are persistent little things that are especially hard to avoid when children share shower facilities and other common areas in gyms and sports arenas.

Fortunately, many effective powders and ointments are available over-the-counter, without a doctor's prescription. They help relieve itching, promote drying and often clear the condition. But if signs and symptoms of a fungal infection continue, the child should be seen by his or her doctor.

See also: YEAST INFECTION.

G

Gas, unusual or excessive

A group of symptoms and signs that includes the frequent burping of air, the passage of intestinal gas, sometimes accompanied by abdominal cramping, and possibly some ABDOMINAL BLOATING.

Infants are prone to excessive gas because, while taking milk, they tend to swallow air while vigorously sucking and gulping. If the air is not completely burped out, it forms bubbles that make their way through the digestive tract, causing cramping as it goes.

For the infant who is having particular problems with gassiness, prevention can be achieved with frequent burping—after every ounce or two fed from a bottle, or every five to ten minutes during breast-feeding. Once the condition exists, you can try placing the baby on its abdomen on top of a heating pad or hot water bottle—taking care to avoid burns. Stimulating the rectum with a lubricated thermometer or a glycerin suppository may facilitate passage of gas.

As the child grows and the diet expands, foods high in nitrogen content may cause excessive gas. Cabbage and beans are notorious offenders. Some older children may develop the habit of swallowing air or may do so when they are anxious.

MILK ALLERGY or intolerance to lactose (milk sugar) may cause excess amounts of gas to be formed. MALABSORPTION SYNDROME can result in gassiness because food is inadequately digested. Cramping, bloody diarrhea, and excessive gassiness may be symptoms of other diseases; a medical evaluation is necessary to arrive at an accurate diagnosis and plan appropriate treatment.

Gastroenteritis

A general term meaning inflammation of the stomach and intestinal tract, especially the small intestine. When an exact infectious cause is determined, the signs and symptoms of the infection are given specific names, such as AMEBIC DYSENTERY or BACILLARY DYSENTERY. Sometimes food poisoning or taking toxic chemicals can cause gastroenteritis; various tropical diseases can also play a role.

Generally speaking, gastroenteritis may be thought of as infectious diarrhea. It may be caused by viruses, bacteria, protozoa, fungi or worms.

Viral gastroenteritis tends to be rather mild and usually clears up in a few days. Bacterial gastroenteritis is more serious. It is marked by the very sudden development of severe diarrhea, which sometimes may be bloody. Vomiting and fever are typical; delirium and symptoms of shock from poisoning are less common, but they may occur.

Any type of gastroenteritis can be extremely dangerous to infants because of the chance of DEHYDRATION, which can occur very quickly, although the time can vary from child to child. Hospitalization—so that fluids can be replaced intravenously and the child can be monitored—is generally necessary. In fact, any child who has lost more than 10 percent of his or her weight because of fluid loss should probably be hospitalized.

Less severe dehydration can be treated at home by restricting solids and milk and placing the child on a clear liquid diet until the condition clears and the doctor approves a gradual reintroduction of solid foods. Parents should understand that a liquid diet means *lots* of liquids. Children need around 4½ ounces of fluid for each 2¼ pounds of body weight. A 30-pound child will therefore require somewhat more than two quarts of clear fluid each day. This diet can be varied by using weakened tea, different fruit juices, water and even carbonated beverages if your child's doctor approves. The most ideal replacment is with one of the commercially balanced electrolyte solutions such as Pedialyte or Lytren, as the child's doctor recommends.

Parents should keep in mind that antispasmodics, antidiarrheal medicines and preparations that stop vomiting may mask symptoms of dehydration or other serious illnesses. These medicines should never be given to infants and small children unless a physician is carefully supervising the youngsters.

German measles

See RUBELLA.

Gilles de la Tourette's syndrome

See TOURETTE'S SYNDROME.

Growth failure

A deviation from a predictable pattern of growth. A child's own, individual previous growth rate is more valuable than statistical comparisons with other children of similar ages. Some children may simply be shorter than others, particularly if their parents are not tall, since genetic influences play a major role in determining height. As long as children do not fall too far from their established pattern, there is no cause for concern.

Infants grow very rapidly in their first year of life. In the first six months they generally double their birth weight and in the next six months, triple it. At the end of the first year, they will have grown about ten inches. Afterward the pattern slows. Each year will generally add about five pounds in weight and about two and one half inches in height. During adolescence a growth spurt occurs, with as much as six to eight inches added height.

If parents have maintained good records and note that a child has definitely slowed in his or her normal growth pattern, medical advice should be sought. A THYROID DISORDER or some other hormonal imbalance may be at fault. Certain illnesses may interfere with growth, but when they are treated appropriately the child can catch up. Above all, parents should avoid forcing extra calories or searching for appealing appetite stimulants. It is generally healthier to be too thin than too fat—unless, of course, the thinness reflects some dangerous disorder, such as ANOREXIA NERVOSA or a malignancy.

Growing pains

Once ascribed to children's vivid imaginations, it is now thought that these joint and muscle pains are probably related to the growth and changing composition of muscles. Some children experience marked discomfort in the arms or legs just with normal play, although the pain is heightened by strenuous exercise such as engaging in sports. Rest, warm baths, the application of heat and the use of mild painkillers such as children's doses of aspirin usually offer some relief.

If there is no joint swelling, no fever, no muscle weakness, no local tenderness when the muscles are pressed, and no weight loss, a doctor's care is probably not needed.

Gynecomastia

Abnormal enlargement of one or both male breasts.

Almost one-half of adolescent boys experience some degree of this condition at some point after puberty. The breast may be tender at times, and there may be some enlargement of the nipples. No medical treatment is needed, for the condition is harmless and disappears of its own accord within a year, or two years at most. However, the situation is apt to cause the adolescent enormous embarrassment, and parental reassurance in addition to a doctor's reassurance may prove helpful.

Only in the rarest of instances does the overdeveloped breast tissue fail to recede; then, if the growth is excessive and a cause for emotional distress that cannot be otherwise resolved, surgical removal may be indicated.

H

Hair, loss and thinning

Loss of hair from any hairy part of the body is technically called alopecia. There are many kinds of alopecia. Here we are concerned only with the loss and thinning of scalp hair.

Hair growth occurs in cycles. During one of the cycles in this process, it is normal for the human scalp to lose from fifty to a hundred hairs each day. Some of this loss may be noticed during combing or brushing, but usually it simply falls away unnoticed and will be replaced by new hair. (Your child is not going bald!)

"Plucking" may contribute to hair loss. Some children—often those given to habits such as thumb sucking—may pull and pluck at the scalp until hair shafts are broken and a baldish spot appears. This is often done unconsciously; when the pulling stops, the hair grows back naturally. Similar bald spots may result from too much traction from barrettes or tight ponytails, or when infants lie on their backs for most of the day.

Certain fever-producing illnesses as well as emotional stress, injuries and adolescents' crash diets may interrupt normal hair growth cycles. But if the precipitating cause is not repeated, a full head of hair will return over a period of several weeks. (Actually only about one-quarter of the total number of hairs fall out, but the loss can be quite noticeable.)

A condition thought to be related to the body's immune system may cause very sudden hair loss in well-outlined patches. Cortisone compounds can speed hair regrowth, but even though these medications can be obtained without a doctor's prescription, they should not be used until a physician diagnoses the problem and recommends such treatment.

Halitosis

See BREATH ODOR.

Hallucinations

A sensed experience of sights, sounds or smells not actually present, but which seem quite real to the person who perceives them.

Hallucinations may occur with high fevers, but they clear and are forgotten once the child's temperature returns to normal. They are caused by increased activity of the nervous system, an effect that drugs such as LSD and mescaline and severe emotional disturbances such as the psychoses share.

Children may seem to have hallucinations in NIGHTMARES AND NIGHT TERRORS. Actually they are experiencing nothing more than dreams, however bad they may be. Parents should also not confuse imagination with hallucinations. IMAGINARY FRIENDS are not hallucinations; they are part of children's rich fantasy life.

Hay fever

Usually a seasonal ALLERGY that strikes in spring, summer, or fall, when airborne pollen is prevalent. The name is misleading. Fever does not occur, and the signs and symptoms result from sensitivity to many wind-borne pollens from trees, grasses, and weeds. Hay fever, also known by the medical term of allergic rhinitis, can be caused by exposure to indoor allergens that are inhaled, such as house dust, feathers, and animal hair.

The symptoms and signs of hay fever can occur suddenly or develop gradually. An early indication may be intense itching of the nose, throat and roof of the mouth. This is followed or accompanied by sneezing, watering of the eyes (which sometimes become red and itchy), and a discharge of clear, thin fluid from the nose. Nasal congestion, when the lining of the nose swells, makes breathing difficult. When the pollen count is particularly high, the air tubes of the lungs may be involved, so that the child has brief, asthmalike attacks with wheezing.

Children who suffer badly from hay fever should see a doctor. When a specific type of pollen is identified as the allergen, it may be possible to desensitize the child through a series of injections that will stimulate the body to produce an immune response. This treatment should begin at least three to four months before the start of the hay fever season. This kind of treatment is undertaken, however, only if the symptoms are very severe.

Milder forms of hay fever can often be dramatically relieved by taking antihistamines. Some of these drugs are available over the counter, but more potent ones can be obtained with a doctor's prescription. Parents should be sure—as with all drugs given to children—that label instructions are followed very carefully.

Headache

Headaches are not rare in children. It is rare, however, that they signal any serious disease.

Nonetheless, it is helpful to a doctor, and ultimately to the child, if parents make notes about their child's complaints of headaches. Is the discomfort localized or diffuse? Is it one-sided? Where did it begin? Is there anything that seemed to bring it on? How long does it last? How often do they occur? At what time of the day does it tend to come on? Is there a family history of similar headaches? And, of particular importance, are there other signs or symptoms present, such as vomiting?

Migraine headaches may occur at any time during childhood or adolescence. A strong family background makes the diagnosis more likely. Migraines tend to occur suddenly and sometimes are preceded by the sensation of lights flashing or there being wavy lines in front of the eyes. The pain is severe and throbbing and is often confined to one side of the head. Nausea and vomiting are fairly common. Children affected just want to lie down in a dark room and be left alone, which is good therapy, since sleep often takes the headache away. A physician's evaluation is needed in order to determine the best course of drug treatment. Parents can help the child understand that he or she may have these headaches off and on throughout life, but that they are not serious.

Tension headaches are seen in younger children but are more prevalent in adolescents. The pain arises from fatigue and/or stress, usually starting in the muscles in the back of the neck, then proceeding upward along each side to the forehead. The pain is dull and aching, and may worsen as the day progresses. There is no vomiting or other symptoms except perhaps for irritability. Aspirin generally offers relief, and sleep seems to clear the headache altogether.

Along with muscle aching, a headache may be an early feature of influenza or other VIRAL INFECTIONS. But contrary to popular opinion, eyestrain and a need for corrective lens are not associated with headaches. Children with SINUSITIS or who are suffering from DEPRESSION or other emotional problems may complain of headaches.

Possibly because headaches are not very common in children, parents often tend to think the worst if their child gets a headache. The fear of brain tumor seems to be high on the list. However, this condition, although ranking high in incidence of childhood tumors, is really quite rare. Headaches caused by tumors are a result of increased pressure within the skull. As the pressure increases, so does vomiting, which may be projectile, that is, the material may shoot out in an arc. Obviously medical attention is necessary, but fortunately, very few parents ever encounter this situation.

Severe headache may also accompany other medical conditions such as SEIZURE DISORDERS or the emergency illnesses MENINGITIS and ENCEPHALITIS. Both meningitis and encephalitis are associated with fever, vomiting, and a stiff neck, serious signs that alert parents to the need for quick medical attention.

Head banging

Impacting the head against any surface, such as when infants sometimes rock against the crib mattress. It apparently provides rhythmic relaxation as they are going to sleep. In an older child, head banging may be an attempt to relive the early security of the crib.

Children rarely persist in the behavior after they reach the age of four, although some continue it into the early school years. Providing an air of relaxation at bedtime may help. Under no circumstances should the child be physically restrained.

Head injury

The heavy, bony casing of the skull is normally an efficient protector of the delicate brain inside it. Unless the skull is severely fractured, the bone acts as a barrier between penetrating wounds and soft nerve tissue. However, the skull cannot prevent the brain from being affected by CONCUSSION when the head is jolted.

Any fairly serious blow to the head is an immediate alarm to call for medical help. If there is any likelihood of a fractured neck or spine, it is best to leave the child in the position in which he or she was found. If the victim is unconscious, protect the airway by gently clearing any fluid in the mouth before it obstructs breathing. Otherwise, try not to move the child until medical personnel arrive. If circumstances are such that the child must be moved, do so with extreme caution. Sometimes gently lifting the body onto a hard surface, such as a wooden plank, provides protection against further movement as the child is being transported to an emergency facility. Any slight bleeding from the ear or nose or bruising around the eye should be regarded as potentially serious signs.

A very severe blow that damages the skull may cause compression of the brain. Pieces of broken bone may press against the brain's surface. The general swelling that accompanies any fracture, which can show on the surface as a puffy area of scalp or skin, can also cause inside swelling that presses against brain tissue. Finally, any bleeding inside the skull will compress the jellylike brain within the hard, bony casing into which it fits so closely.

If the compression is severe enough, it can cause unconsciousness and even death. Unlike the instant knockout of a concussion, unconsciousness develops gradually in cases of compression. The child may pass through stages of headache, irritability, nausea and vomiting, and make uncontrolled jerky movements before becoming drowsy and losing consciousness. This may take minutes or hours, depending on how much and how fast pressure is building.

Although any forceful blow to the head, particularly if followed by a period of unconsciousness, must be considered a true medical emergency, parents should be relieved to know that children have a remarkable ability to recover from what seems to be, and often is, a very serious head injury.

When a head injury occurs, certain precautions should be followed. The child may be allowed to sleep, but should be awakened every two hours and checked for the symptoms listed here:

1. Nonuse of an arm or leg
2. Inequality in the size of the pupils of the eyes
3. Vomiting
4. Unusual behavior
5. Difficulty in arousing the child

Should any of these problems be present, the child must be examined at a medical facility.

Hearing loss

Parents can usually determine whether a child has a hearing problem by certain patterns of behavior (for example, the child's seeming to ignore noise or showing an unusually limited attention span); by difficulties a toddler encounters trying to speak; or by simple tests such as measuring the distance at which the child can hear a whisper or a watch ticking. Specialized testing is necessary to determine the extent of hearing loss and the range of frequencies that can be heard. One method of testing, called speech audiometry, uses a recording of spoken words played through headphones at varying degrees of loudness. This method has an advantage over the tone method (tones versus words) because it permits the tester to determine more precisely if the hearing problem is caused by conductive DEAFNESS or nerve deafness. Speech audiometry also allows an assessment of the value a hearing aid might provide to the child.

In the United States it is fairly standard practice to provide free hearing tests to children of school age, especially when they are in kindergarten or first grade. If a hearing problem is discovered, parents should immediately seek outside professional assistance for the child.

Deafness, if present, is a particularly serious problem in the child's development and education. Children need to be able to communicate their feelings and thoughts and to be able to share in the experiences of others. Many countries have schools for the deaf that specialize in the teaching of language and of lip reading, together with other methods of communication such as finger spelling and other forms of sign language.

It is generally accepted, however, that the successful development of skills in lip and speech reading is much more important than sign language. Heavy dependence on sign language may lead the child to withdraw gradually from social involvement with those whose hearing is normal.

Heartburn

See INDIGESTION.

Heart murmurs

Abnormal sounds heard by a physician listening to the heart with a stethoscope. A *functional* murmur is absolutely harmless, in medical language. But on occasion a murmur may signify some defect in the heart or its valves, *organic* in technical terminology.

Functional murmurs are quite common in children. They are caused by turbulence in the blood as it flows through the heart. Approximately 15 to 20 percent of the population have such murmurs, and they live full and active lives without a need for any medical or surgical treatment to correct the murmur. Functional murmurs do not lead to heart disease and many of them go away spontaneously as the child gets older.

Even organic murmurs that do indicate some heart abnormality do not generally cause any limitation of activity. Regularly scheduled physical examinations permit the doctor to monitor the situation and detect problems before they become major. Sometimes antibiotics will be prescribed to prevent infections should any operations or major dental procedures be done.

In addition to the physician's physical examination, several diagnostic tests are used to investigate the heart. The electrocardiogram, or EKG, makes a tracing of heart activity. Chest X rays will indicate whether the heart may be enlarged. The echocardiogram uses sound waves to depict the way the heart is working. In cardiac catheterization, a dye is injected so that specialists can actually see how the heart is functioning. The results of these tests help the doctor prescribe the correct course of treatment.

See also: HOLE IN THE HEART.

Heart rate

The hearts of infants and children beat much faster than the average 70 times a minute that is normal for adults.

Newborn babies have an average heart rate of 120 to 140; during bouts of crying or excessive activity this may increase to about 170 or more, whereas in sleep it drops to between 70 and 90.

As the child grows older, the rate slows. By four to six years of age, the heart rate is about 100 per minute; by the age of eight to ten, it drops to an average of 90. It reaches adult levels by late adolescence.

Parents should keep in mind that these are *averages.* For example, a six-year-old may have a heart rate as low as 75 or as high as 115 and still be within normal range. Also, from about twelve to eighteen, girls will tend to have heart rates approximately five points higher than boys.

Just as in adults, heart rate will be affected by strenuous activity, excitement, fear and various other emotional states, as well as by certain drugs and foods or drinks such as excessive coffee drinking and cigarette smoking. It is only when children over eight or ten years old consistently show a heart rate of 120 or more that parents should arrange for a medical examination to determine whether there is some serious underlying cause for the fast beating.

Heat rash

Technically known as miliaria, heat rash or prickly heat refers to a skin inflammation in which pinpoint blisters progress to a bright red, dotted appearance. In severe cases the spots seem to join into one large rash.

Heat rash occurs when excessive heat or too-heavy clothing cause a blockage of the sweat glands. Infants are particularly prone because of the immaturity of their skin structure. The cheeks, neck, trunk and diaper areas are commonly involved.

The condition is not harmful, and there is no specific treatment. Parents should avoid overdressing babies when the weather is hot. Cool baths and the application of a light medicated powder may reduce the irritation, and the child may be more comfortable in an air-conditioned or air-cooled environment. Prevention of prickly heat involves avoiding high temperatures and humidity, keeping out of direct sunlight, and dressing in porous, nonbinding clothes.

Heat stroke and heat exhaustion

An acute illness resulting from prolonged exposure to high environmental temperatures such as may be experienced in a closed and improperly ventilated car; an abandoned refrigerator; or a closet or other tightly enclosed space.

Heat exhaustion or heat stroke happens like this: In an attempt to maintain normal body temperature, the child sweats excessively causing a loss of body fluids and salts. The child appears pale, and the skin is cold and clammy. Beads of perspiration may appear on the forehead. Shallow breathing is usually present, and sometimes the child vomits or feels like vomiting. Confusion is an early sign. Left unattended, the child lapses into unconsciousness.

As soon as the situation is discovered, remove the child to a cool place. Place the youngster on his or her back with the head lowered and the feet elevated. Cover the child with a blanket and phone an emergency medical unit for help. If conscious, children with heat stroke may be given short sips of salt water (one teaspoonful of salt to one pint of water).

Compare SUNSTROKE.

Hemangioma

Small benign, not malignant, tumors that are among the most common congenital defects seen in children. They affect the vascular system and appear as a disorganized collection of small blood vessels, usually in a well-circumscribed area. Hemangiomas may occur in any organ of the body, but they are usually found on the skin.

By far the commonest of the hemangiomas is the "salmon patch." This irregular, reddened, flat area on the forehead or the upper eyelids will appear in up to 40 percent of all newborn babies. Many infants will also have similar marks on the back of the scalp and the nape of the neck. The overwhelming majority of these marks will spontaneously disappear by the time the child is one year old; no treatment is necessary. Occasionally the patches will be noticeable later in life whenever the child cries or is flushed. But there is no real disfigurement.

The "strawberry hemangioma" is a raised, red-to-purple mass that develops during the first few months of life; it may be noticeable at birth. It starts out as a tiny red spot anywhere on the body but usually on the face, neck, or trunk. Over the first six months of life, the strawberry mark enlarges rapidly; most of them reach their final size by the time the child is one year old. Some "strawberries" may reach two to three inches across, raised from one-half to one inch from the skin, before they stop growing. Then, for several months, the size may remain stable. But as the mass outgrows its own blood supply, it begins to whiten and shrink in size. Most of these hemangiomas are gone by the time the child is three years old; all that remains is a faint discoloration of the skin or, in some cases, no mark at all. Very large hemangiomas, for example, those that may cover an entire half of the child's face, may take longer to go away. Ordinarily no treatment is required, and parents can rest assured that their child is not disfigured for life. Only if a vital organ such as the eye is involved need special medical attention be undertaken. Occasionally the center of the hemangioma will ooze and crust as it breaks down. If that happens, infection could set in, and an antibiotic cream may be needed.

The "cavernous hemangioma" is a tangled mass of blood vessels; it tends to lie deeper in the skin. The tumor has an irregular border and a soft, bubbly consistency. Many are noticed at birth, but some will not become evident until the baby is a few months old. Sometimes a purplish discoloration is all that is seen; sometimes the mass sticks up from the skin's surface. They grow slower than strawberry hemangiomas, and they take longer to go away if, indeed, they do go away. However, because of their depth, there is usually no disfiguration and no treatment is needed unless some vital organ is affected.

"Port wine stains" are pink-to-red flat marks that usually occur on the face. They vary in size and have irregular borders. Port wine stains grow as the child grows and, unlike strawberry marks and cavernous hemangiomas, they do not go away spontaneously. In the past, treatment has not been very satisfactory. Current therapy that involves use of an argon laser beam is showing some promising results. The procedure lightens the port wine stain considerably, but it is not recommended for children younger than nine. A few cosmetic companies have specialized in devising bases and coverups that make the mark much less noticeable.

Hemophilia

An inherited disease in which the blood fails to clot within the time range generally considered normal. It can result in severe and life-threatening bleeding unless the patient receives immediate medical treatment.

Hemophilia is a genetic disease that affects males, but the defect is carried by females who are generally symptomless. The defect involves abnormalities in the blood-clotting factor, which can be diagnosed by laboratory tests that reveal functional defects and a lowered quantity of clotting factor. A carrier has about a fifty-fifty chance of passing the disease to her daughters, who will themselves be carriers with an equal chance of passing on the disease. A male hemophiliac cannot pass on the disease to his sons, but all his daughters will be carriers since the disease is sex-linked to the X chromosome in body cells.

The disorder may be noticed very early, for example, with excessive bleeding at circumcision, or, especially in milder forms, it may not become evident until the boy has a tooth extracted or has other minor surgery. Often a minor scrape or cut will cause abnormal bleeding, and the hemophiliac may show large and deep-seated bruises as a result of extremely minor injuries that other children incur almost daily without difficulty.

The disease can be managed by infusion of a substance called cryoprecipitate. This material is prepared by adding the clotting factor to plasma that is quick-frozen, then slow-thawed.

Hemophilia is rare. It is estimated that there are approximately 25,000 hemophiliacs in the United States—which means an incidence of only one in 10,000. However, without parental understanding of what the disease means and without appropriate treatment, boys with hemophilia can literally bleed to death or develop crippling deformities from blood seeping into body joints. Parents can actively participate in their child's therapy by learning how to infuse cryoprecipitate at home. Should bleeding occur at an easily accessible body area, applying direct hand pressure or elastic bandages can usually control the bleeding until the child reaches the doctor's office or an emergency medical facility. Other drugs may be prescribed that will lessen bleeding in the case of dental extraction or minor surgery.

Counseling may be of great benefit. Both the parents and the affected child need support in their efforts to maintain as normal a life-style as is possible. Also, some parents may want to review their plans to have additional children in light of the risk of transmitting hemophilia.

Hepatitis

Inflammation of the liver, most commonly caused by VIRAL INFECTIONS.

Infectious hepatitis was thought to be transmitted solely by drinking water or milk or by eating food contaminated with infected human feces, for example, where poor sewage facilities exist. Serum hepatitis was thought to be transmitted solely by using contaminated blood in transfusions or through injections with contaminated needles or syringes. It is now known that both forms of viral hepatitis, now often called hepatitis A and hepatitis B, can be transmitted by either route, though one generally predominates.

Hepatitis A, also known as infectious hepatitis or short-term hepatitis, is the more common form in children. It is most often transmitted by the feces-to-mouth route, but the disease is highly contagious. If the child has been around a hepatitis patient, parents should contact a doctor and inquire about the advisability of gamma globulin injections as a preventative measure.

The incubation period is generally from about two weeks to seven weeks. Children may becomes listless or cranky, but home treatment, mostly consisting of bed rest and/or restriction of activity, is usually possible. Because of the contagiousness of the disease, other family members and close contacts should be given preventative injections of gamma globulin.

Hepatitis B, also called serum hepatitis or long-incubation

hepatitis, is potentially the more serious form of viral hepatitis. The incubation period may last from around seven to twenty-six weeks after exposure to infection, usually through contaminated needles or syringes or a contaminated blood transfusion. When the child has been transfused, this information alerts the physician to suspect hepatitis as he or she does a diagnostic workup.

Early symptoms of hepatitis B often resemble those of influenza. The urine may appear dark, and the stools frequently take on a grayish color. Other indications typically include a general feeling of malaise (a vague sense of being unwell), fever and later development of JAUNDICE. However, jaundice may not appear, especially in those who have had a previous infection and have developed at least partial immunity. The child usually has no appetite and is apt to become weak and drowsy. In severe cases hospitalization may be needed, especially if intravenous solutions of glucose (sugar) are needed to compensate for DEHYDRATION.

Once the child has hepatitis, no specific drug therapy is effective. However, the outlook for full recovery is very favorable. Even a severely damaged liver has a remarkable capacity for regeneration and recovery.

Hernia

A hernia may occur at any site in the body, as, for example, a herniated vertebral disk (a slipped disk). It simply means that some piece of body tissue has ruptured through an opening and is sticking out from whatever structure normally confines it.

Children most often suffer from umbilical hernias or inguinal (groin) hernias. An umbilical hernia is a bulge beneath the area where the umbilical cord was attached. Sometimes while the baby is still in the uterus, cord tissues fail to close. Umbilical hernias are more common in girls than in boys, and in black children more so than in whites.

Although occasionally an infant will have a bulge as large as an orange, most umbilical hernias are small, becoming more noticeable when the baby cries. There is no pain. The bulge usually consists of intestine and supporting structures that protrude through the opening in the abdominal wall. This is, of course, all inside. What you see on the baby's abdomen is simply a skin-covered bulge that tends to recede under slight pressure.

Some controversy lingers about the usefulness of strapping with "belly binders," but it is generally thought that these measures do not help and may possibly do harm. No treatment is required; most umbilical hernias recede by themselves by the time the child is one or two, although it may take until about age five if the bulge is unusually large. Surgery should be avoided unless some complication, such as pain or intestinal blockage, has occurred.

Inguinal hernias may appear at any time of life. Most often a portion of the intestinal tract slides in and out of the scrotum. Less commonly, intestinal material protrudes directly through the abdominal wall and into the groin area—a defect that can be seen in girls as well as boys. Like umbilical hernias, they usually arise because certain tissues did not close properly when the fetus was developing; an opening remains through which the intestine bulges out.

Inguinal hernias are usually discovered in babies as a bulge alongside the penis or in the scrotum itself. In girls, the mass will appear in the groin area alongside the external genitals.

A particular problem is incarceration, that is, when the hernia slides, gets locked in and is unable to move. Pain, irritability, problems with bowel movements and pressure may develop. If swelling in the loop of the bowel occurs, an INTESTINAL OBSTRUCTION will develop and the hernia is said to be strangulated. Emergency surgery is necessary. Otherwise an inguinal hernia can normally wait for elective surgery, although it probably should be done as soon as it can be conveniently scheduled. When diagnosed in a very young infant the procedure can be deferred until the baby is older and surgical risks are diminished. Parents should bear in mind, however, that if any bulge is hard, if pain is present, or if symptoms such as vomiting and ABDOMINAL BLOATING are present, emergency medical treatment should be sought immediately.

On rare occasions an infant will be born with a diaphragmatic hernia, where abdominal contents poke through an abnormal opening that exists in the diaphragm, the large muscle sheet that separates the abdominal and chest spaces. The baby will have trouble breathing, and immediate surgery must be performed. In other instances, when the defect is very small, it takes days for trouble to occur. Whenever a diaphragmatic hernia is discovered, the infant is treated with various emergency procedures to assist breathing before and after the surgery.

Herpangina

A viral illness characterized by small ulcers in the mouth and on the gums, with fevers as high as 105°F. The infection lasts for up to three or four days and then goes away by itself. No active treatment is necessary, but the parent can offer the child some relief by giving cool liquids, a fever-reducer such as aspirin, and perhaps by dabbing the sores with a cotton swab dipped in an astringent mouthwash. Parents should also watch for any signs of DEHYDRATION if the infant or child absolutely refuses to drink.

Herpes simplex (Type I)

An infectious disease caused by a virus of the same name. It is often referred to merely as herpes, but it should not be confused with the totally separate disease known as HERPES ZOSTER, commonly known as shingles, or with herpes simplex Type II, which causes genital infections in adults.

The disorder is marked by the formation of groups of small cold sores or fever blisters at the corners of the mouth, ocular herpes (blisters around the eyes), or occasionally on other parts of the body.

No specific treatment exists, although recently special antiviral creams have been developed that may help control the severity and extent of the lesions.

Herpes zoster

Herpes zoster, commonly known as shingles, is rare in children, although it sometimes occurs when the chickenpox virus, lying dormant since a mild episode of that common disease, is reactivated. The disease is usually mild in children, and the outlook for full recovery is very good.

The virus typically attacks the roots of sensory nerves just outside the spinal cord. Since it usually affects one nerve or group of nerves, the eruption of red rash and blisters generally occurs on only one side of the body, for example, one side of the face, one shoulder or arm or along one side of the chest or abdomen.

No specific treatment exists, although children may be given childhood doses of aspirin or acetaminophen for relief of pain if that becomes a problem.

Herpetic stomatitis

An acute inflammation and blistering inside the mouth caused by the herpes virus. The child may run temperatures as high as 104° or 105°F for a week to ten days. Intense mouth discomfort may cause a child to refuse to eat, and irritability is common.

The disease clears up by itself, without complications, and no treatment is necessary. Applying cotton swabs dipped in an astringent mouthwash may offer some relief, as will cool liquids and aspirin or aspirinlike fever reducers given in children's doses.

Although this infection is caused by a herpes virus, it is *not* the same one as is transmitted sexually.

Hiccups

A forceful body reflex resulting from a spasm of the diaphragm, the thin muscle sheet that separates the abdominal and chest cavities. The sound made is characteristic, and from it comes the name. Hiccups tend to occur when the diaphragm or the nerves that supply it are subjected to pressure or irritation.

Infants often swallow air with feedings, which causes the stomach to increase in size, squeezing the diaphragm. Vigorous sucking and overfeeding make the problem worse. Frequent burping can help keep the stomach from distending too much. Older children may get hiccups from eating too rapidly or swallowing large quantities of carbonated beverages.

More serious medical conditions may be responsible, such as infections of the abdominal cavity, kidney failure, or a perforated ulcer. But if such a process is underway, there will be other symptoms far more dramatic than hiccups. In most instances of ordinary hiccups, no treatment is required. Many home remedies (drinking water with the head held forward and down, raising one's arms, and holding one's breath, etc.) exist.

But scaring a child is definitely not recommended. Only in the rarest of instances does prolonged hiccuping, which can become quite exhausting, necessitate medical attention.

Hip dislocation

Some babies are born with an abnormally lax hip joint, that is, it is abnormally mobile, and the knobby portion of bone slides easily in and out of its socket. In some instances a dislocation can accidentally be caused during breech birth.

In most cases this difficulty will be spotted within a few weeks and treatment, often with a splint or a specially padded diaper, is started immediately.

Hips that are not properly joined at birth are likely to become progressively less stable as the child grows. Hip joints weak at birth may not become truly dislocated for several months. Parents may be able to recognize the condition if one of the baby's legs seems slightly shorter than the other, or if unusual wrinkling of the skin exists on one of the child's thighs or buttocks. It is important to bring this to the attention of a physician, because the sooner a hip dislocation is noted, the easier it can be treated medically, without recourse to surgery.

Hip pain

Pain in or around the hip joint is uncommon in childhood. However, hip pain can occur, most often as a result of twisting falls that strain the joint and the muscles around it. Rest and elevating the leg will facilitate healing, and appropriate children's dosages of aspirin or similar painkillers will relieve the initial discomfort.

Often the child does not complain of pain but merely limps, thereby protecting the affected side. An infant or toddler may refuse to bear weight when held up.

Boys between the ages of four and ten seem to be susceptible to a condition known as Perthes' disease. For unknown reasons, the top part of the long thigh bone becomes fragmented. Treatment, imperative if the hip joint is to continue to develop properly, consists of rest and bracing so that the extremity is positioned in a way that allows some weight bearing without further stressing the diseased bone. Therapy may take several years, but results are good, allowing for normal joint development.

Teenagers who gain weight rapidly or who are overweight to start with may develop a condition in which the portion of bone that acts as a center of growth slips from its normal location at the head of the thigh bone. This occurs slowly, and knee pain may occur before hip discomfort develops. X rays will show slippage, and immobilization by cast or surgery is required to halt progression of the disorder.

Other medical conditions can cause hip pain. Bacterial infection, characterized also by fever, may affect the hip joint. Bacterial infection is a serious condition requiring emergency medical care if the joint is to be preserved. An inflammation of the hip joint, called synovitis, may also accompany or follow certain viral infections. No long-term complications follow this disorder, but medical evaluation is needed to differentiate it from results of a bacterial infection. JUVENILE RHEUMATOID ARTHRITIS, as well as benign or malignant tumors, tuberculosis and other unusual infections may cause hip pain.

Hives

A skin reaction, known by the medical name of urticaria, that shows localized swellings or elevations of the skin that are red and intensely itchy.

Occasionally hives are associated with viral infections (especially in younger children) or urinary tract infections and strep throat. However, by far the commonest cause is allergy. Hypersensitivity to a wide variety of substances causes histamine to "pour out" within the body, resulting in an accumulation of fluid in the skin or mucous membranes. Therefore, doctors will generally prescribe antihistamines, although other approaches (special inhalants or medicines that thin mucus accumulations) are sometimes used.

Cold compresses may offer some home treatment relief. If an underlying infection is present, it must be treated with antibiotics.

Compare ALLERGY.

Hoarseness

A raspy quality of the voice or breathing pattern. During childhood the commonest reason for hoarseness is an acute infection such as CROUP or LARYNGITIS. If they are associated with breathing difficulties, these illnesses require emergency medical care. When breathing is not affected, providing moisturized air with vaporizers or bathroom steam and plenty of fluids will help lessen symptoms.

Hoarseness may come from voice overuse. Children tend to be noisy; extended periods of loud play or screaming may cause them to be hoarse. Even with normal voice use, children may tire their vocal cords. Rest and quiet cures the problem. Hoarsening that develops slowly and becomes progressively worse could indicate a papilloma or singer's nodes, little nonmalignant tumors that usually recede without surgical removal. Occasionally newborn infants have a softening of the supporting structures around the vocal cords, or one cord may be paralyzed. Neither of these disorders causes any long-term problem, and the difficulty is usually outgrown.

Hole in the heart

A congenital (present-at-birth) malformation in which a septal defect permits abnormal flow of blood from one heart chamber to another.

The two upper chambers, called atria, are separated by a membranous wall called the atrial septum. Incomplete development allows an atrial septal defect or hole. The thick and muscular bottom chambers that pump blood out into the body, called ventricles, are separated by another septum. Incomplete development here creates a ventricular septal defect or hole.

Because a hole in the heart disrupts the normal passage of blood through the heart, the baby does not get enough oxygen circulated and may look bluish in color.

Diagnosis, now frequently made soon after birth, depends on physical findings, chest X rays, heart tracings done by the electrocardiograph, and, if indicated, a heart catheterization. The latter test involves the injection of a dye directly into the bloodstream while special heart X rays are taken. Treatment, either medical or surgical, depends on the degree of symptoms and the extent of the heart abnormality. Parents should be reassured that current medical practice allows increasingly successful treatment with minimal or no remaining disability.

Hodgkin's disease

A disorder in which there is a painless overgrowth of lymphatic glands throughout the body; red blood corpuscles are reduced in number, so that severe anemia develops; and internal organs such as the spleen become enlarged.

Although Hodgkin's disease often strikes in young adulthood, it also affects children, boys more often than girls. It is sometimes confused with leukemia; in fact, one of its technical names is pseudoleukemia. However, it appears not to be neoplastic (a true cancer), and it is not marked by the overwhelming increase in white blood cells found in leukemia.

Lymphatic enlargement may occur first in the neck, then the armpits and the groin, and finally inside the deep internal glands and organs. There is little if any pain, but fever, HERPES ZOSTER, a bronze discoloration and profound weakness are common.

Aggressive medical treatment with modern drugs or X-ray therapy offers some relief from symptoms, and remissions of several years are not uncommon. However, the disease remains a very serious one for which no permanent cure is yet known. Therefore family counseling may help the parents, siblings, and the sufferer come to terms with this illness.

Compare LEUKEMIA.

Homosexual behavior

The preference of an individual for sexual contact and/or romantic involvement with members of the same sex.

Since at least occasional homosexual behavior is seen in many species, and because preteens frequently form very close attachments with buddies with whom they may engage in a little sexual exploration, authorities used to believe that most older children go through a homosexual stage that they outgrow. However, this seems not always to be the case. Rarely does some crisis in gender identity play a role in a preference for homosexuality. These young people seem quite clear about their maleness or their femaleness, but for reasons that none of the multiple theories has ever conclusively proved, they simply find their affectional needs best fulfilled by persons of the same sex.

For most, the conflict does not surround their homosexuality; rather, it concerns familial and societal responses and worry about how disapproval and not fitting in may interfere with their leading a normal and productive life.

Parents may feel angry, or feel they are at fault. It is important that love prevail and they not abandon their own child. Frank, open, supportive discussions will be helpful to the parents and to the child. Consulting with a physician or other professional should be undertaken *not* as a means of altering the young person's thoughts and feelings but only to make sure that he or she is comfortable in this choice and is fully aware of the implications of swimming against the mainstream. In those instances in which the individual actually wishes to assume a heterosexual life-style, counseling can sometimes be helpful. But parents are cautioned not to be overly optimistic about change. In general, sheer acceptance even if they don't actually understand goes a long way in strengthening family bonds and in helping the child achieve self-respect and balance. Some parents have found supportive groups such as Parents of Gays helpful.

Hornet stings

See STINGS.

Human bites

The human mouth has a remarkable variety and amount of bacterial growth that does no harm there but can cause infections if the microorganisms are driven through a break in the skin. Often this occurs in rough play or from a fist landing on someone's teeth. Depending on the site, a severe and progressive infection can develop. The hands are in special need of prompt treatment because tendons and other important structures may be permanently damaged from an untreated infection.

Whenever skin is broken by contact with teeth, thoroughly cleanse the area with soap and water. Observe carefully for redness or swelling. If these signs develop, or if pus seeps from the wound, seek immediate medical evaluation. Antibiotic therapy is necessary and, in some cases, surgical drainage of the infection may be required. Many physicians feel that any human bite which results in a break in the skin must be treated immediately even before there are any signs of infection.

Small children will sometimes bite playmates or adults out of anger. Biting the child back is not a good way to stop this behavior; neither will a slap on the face teach the child a proper way of handling anger. If you sense that the child is about to bite someone, quickly remove the child from the situation. Discipline might include having the child sit in a chair or go to his or her room to think about the matter in isolation.

Hydrocele

A collection of fluid around a testicle or the cord to the testicle. It is not uncommon in newborns, in whom the scrotal sac on the affected side will appear swollen and tense. It can also be diagnosed by simply passing light from a flashlight through the scrotum.

The fluid will be absorbed by the body and the swelling will disappear, usually within the first year of life. There is no adverse effect and no treatment is necessary.

However, hydroceles that develop later in infancy or after the baby is one year old should be managed differently because of the possibility of an associated HERNIA, for which surgery might be indicated.

Hyperactive behavior

A form of behavior in which a child seems to be constantly moving, and in which a child's activity level is far more excessive than one would expect in children of that age. The term used to be used as a diagnostic category; now hyperactivity is considered to be part of ATTENTION DEFICIT DISORDERS.

Children who are hyperactive will be extremely loud and noisy. Crowded places will stimulate increased levels of purposeless movement. Shopping and visiting become major undertakings, and baby-sitters may refuse to sit with a hyperactive child. Such children climb, run, fidget, and squirm. Teachers report disruptive behavior. Not even sleep is restful; in the morning, bed clothing may be on the floor in a tangled mess.

Understandably, but unfortunately, many hyperactive children are seen as simply misbehaving. They're yelled at and disciplined for something they cannot control, which increases the child's anger at what is perceived as unfair treatment.

The cycle must be broken if the child is to mature properly. But treatment should not be undertaken lightly. A thorough evaluation by a team of medical and psychological professionals is needed. Both medications and environmental changes may be recommended. A relationship to diet and the adverse effects of some food additives may also be found to play a role. In any event, parents are urged to seek help, otherwise learning will be impossible and the child's chances for success as an adult will be severely hampered.

See also: IMPULSIVE BEHAVIOR.

Hypermetropia

See FARSIGHTEDNESS.

Hyperopia

See FARSIGHTEDNESS.

Hypertension

Abnormally high blood pressure is not common in children in the absence of some medical disorder that can be diagnosed and treated. Therefore, parents are urged to seek medical advice if their child is determined, for example, by a school nurse, to have high blood pressure.

See also: BLOOD PRESSURE.
Compare HYPOTENSION.

Hyperthyroidism

See THYROID DISORDER.

Hyperventilation

Breathing too fast and too much.

Children who are hyperventilating may also feel numbness or tingling sensations, a certain amount of weakness or even faintness. Severe episodes may lead to muscle spasms and loss of consciousness, as the body is out of synch because an abnormal amount of carbon dioxide is being breathed out.

Occasionally hyperventilation indicates the presence of some disease, but more often than not it results from anxiety. Once a doctor has determined that there is no disease, children can often be helped merely by understanding that anxiety causes their symptoms and that they can avoid the symptoms by avoiding the anxiety. If this does not work, seek some professional counseling.

The old paper bag trick actually works to treat hyperventilation. Get a paper bag large enough to cover the child's mouth and nose. Hold it very close to the child's face and have him or her breathe into the bag and rebreathe the air in the bag. If the child does this long enough, perhaps several tries of ten times in and ten times out between brief rests, the normal level of carbon dioxide in the bloodstream returns and the symptoms go away.

Medicines should not be used without approval of the child's doctor.

See also: PANIC ATTACK.

Hypoglycemia

An abnormally low level of glucose (sugar) in the circulating blood. The symptoms include nervousness, cold sweats, weakness, a feeling of acute fatigue, irritability, and, in severe and untreated cases, mental disturbances such as confusion, hallucinations, or bizarre behavior. In extreme cases, particularly in a child with DIABETES MELLITUS, untreated hypoglycemia may result in loss of consciousness or even death.

Children with mild episodes respond to orange juice, honey, or other sweet substances. In moderate spells a child also needs carbohydrates that can be absorbed more slowly, such as a banana, apple, bread, or cereals. Children with severe reactions should always be taken to a doctor for evaluation and for more sophisticated care, such as administration of glucagon.

Hypoglycemia is fairly common in newborn infants; approximately four out of every 1,000 full-term babies and about sixteen out of every 1,000 prematures babies have this condition. Prompt medical evaluation and treatment are usually successful in correcting the abnormality.

Hypotension

Abnormally low blood pressure is even more rare in children than HYPERTENSION, occurring mostly in the instance of severe SHOCK, for which emergency medical attention should be sought. Childhood hypotension is so rare that most references fail to list specific guidelines; therefore, if a child is found to have blood pressure readings lower than average, he or she should be checked by a physician.

See also: BLOOD PRESSURE.

Hypothermia

A condition in which the body's temperature drops below its norm. In extreme cases it may drop dramatically and prove fatal.

In very sick or premature infants, in whom the body's metabolic needs create rapid heat loss, isolette temperatures may have to be regulated by hospital staff in order to encourage maintenance of the baby's normal body temperature. Otherwise, hypothermia is very rare in infants and children unless they are subjected to extreme deprivation (e.g., lack of heat and warm clothing) or, for example, they are exposed to freezing temperatures over a prolonged period of time.

Hypothyroidism

See THYROID DISORDERS.

I

Imaginary friends

Companions children create for themselves.

Until they are around the age of four or sometimes older, children have a natural difficulty separating reality from imagination. Unless this confusion permeates most of the child's everyday life, or signs of EMOTIONAL WITHDRAWAL are present, this rich imagination is actually a good thing. It permits a child to test newly learned social skills, communicate certain thoughts and feelings, and boost creative thinking. Even when a child has playmates and siblings, he or she may create a very special friend with whom special moments can be shared.

Parents should never scold or tease the child. At the same time, neither should they go overboard in integrating the imaginary friend into the entire family scene. As long as children understand that this is part of their own "pretend" world, they should be allowed to enjoy their imaginary friend without interference.

Immunization

An attempt to make the body resistant to a disease by injecting a specific substance that in some way prevents or lessens the effects of the disease. In active immunization a vaccine is given that stimulates the body's protective mechanisms to prepare antibodies that fight the disease when it is encountered. Passive immunization is used when an individual has already been exposed to the disease.

It is now routine in the United States and Canada to immunize against MEASLES, MUMPS, RUBELLA (German measles), POLIOMYELITIS, and a triad called DPT: DIPHTHERIA, PERTUSSIS (whooping cough), and TETANUS (lockjaw) along the suggested schedule of vaccination shown on the next page.

Immunization procedures have drastically reduced the deaths and complications from these once lethal diseases. Although some minimal risks are involved, no child should be denied this protection. Parents whose beliefs prohibit the unnecessary introduction of medical substances into children's bodies should give extremely careful consideration to the consequences of exposing nonimmunized children to the germs and viruses they are likely to encounter in everyday life. Of course, if the child has had an IMMUNIZATION REACTION, tends to be allergic, or is already sick, these situations must be discussed with the doctor whenever any immunization is planned.

Age	Immunization
2 months	DPT/oral polio vaccine
4 months	DPT/oral polio vaccine
6 months	DPT/oral polio vaccine (optional)
15 months	Measles, mumps, rubella (MMR)
18 months	DPT/polio boosters
4–6 years	DPT/polio boosters
14–16 years	DT (a special vaccine with tetanus toxoid and a reduced dose of diphtheria vaccine)
Every 10 years	Tetanus booster

Immunization reaction

An adverse effect in someone who has been injected with an IMMUNIZATION material.

By far the vast majority of children experience little or no reaction to the routine series of immunizations. Practicing pediatricians strongly believe that the benefits of protection far outweigh the slight chance of hazard. However, because potentially serious complications can occasionally arise, parents should be aware of these risks. Also, if a child has had *any* adverse reaction to previous immunizations, the doctor should be told. These signs include:

1. Convulsion.
2. Shock.
3. Fever over 104°F.
4. Screaming or crying for more than three hours. When this is a significant sign, the infant or toddler cannot be calmed no matter what is done.
5. Lethargy or sleepiness for more than three hours. The child who falls asleep and is aroused only with great difficulty, even

at feeding time, may have a more serious reaction with the succeeding injection.

CLEARLY, A PARENT SHOULD ALSO CALL THE DOCTOR AT THE TIME WHEN ANY OF THESE SIGNS APPEAR! IMMUNIZATIONS SHOULD NOT BE GIVEN TO THE CHILD WHO HAS AN ACUTE ILLNESS MORE SERIOUS THAN A COLD, AND DISORDERS OF THE NERVOUS SYSTEM MAY RULE AGAINST IMMUNIZATION.

The common childhood immunizations and their possible reactions are:

Oral polio vaccine No immediate side effect is seen. Only one in as many as 8.1 million doses will be associated with development of the disease in the child or in some unimmunized person with whom he or she comes in contact. Permanent crippling or even death may occur. Anyone with an illness that impairs body defense mechanisms should not be given this vaccine.

DPT (DIPHTHERIA, PERTUSSIS [whooping cough], and TETANUS) Most children will have some soreness and even swelling at the injection site. Fevers may occur in the first twenty-four to forty-eight hours, with temperatures of 102° to 103°F.

In about one out of every 7,000 doses given, somewhat more serious side effects may be seen: high fever (temperature over 103°F), convulsions, undue irritability, extreme lethargy, and shock (signaled by paleness, breathing difficulty, unresponsiveness). Much more rarely, permanent brain damage may occur in one out of every 310,000 children immunized. On even rarer occasion, death is a possibility.

MMR (MEASLES, MUMPS, RUBELLA) About 20 percent of children immunized will get a rash or fever ten days to two weeks after immunization. Usually the fever will be low grade, but temperature might reach 103°F. Although it has not been confirmed, it is said that encephalitis (an inflammation of the brain) may occur in one out of every million children who get the measles vaccine (the incidence of encephalitis in an individual who contracts natural measles is one in a thousand).

A mild swelling of the salivary glands along the underside of the jaw may follow a mumps injection, but this clears spontaneously. The rubella vaccine may be followed by aching or swelling of the joints, which is usually noticed two to ten weeks after the injection; the swelling clears in two or three days.

While parents should be aware of these reactions and risks and should be sure to discuss with the physician any previous adverse reactions, they should be reassured that routine immunization has dramatically improved the health of children in the United States. For example, before the pertussis vaccine was used, each year about 265,000 cases of whooping cough occurred with 7,000 deaths. By the early 1980s there were only 1,000 to 3,000 cases with 5 to 20 deaths a year. The disease itself is extremely dangerous because it can cause long-term problems with the lungs or brain and may result in death. Avoidance of immunization is not advised. A lengthy car trip carries a far greater chance of a bad outcome than all the immunizations combined.

Impetigo

Impetigo, technically called pyoderma, is caused when bacteria, usually staphylococci (or staph), enter small breaks in the skin, such as those caused by insect bites or scratching.

It may start as a small area of redness, generally with a blister. As it spreads, by scratching or simply because of the large number of staph present, which may invade other tiny skin breaks, the blisters ooze a yellow fluid that dries to form crusts.

Generally speaking, impetigo can be cured in a few days if treatment is applied vigorously as soon as the condition is noticed. The child should be bathed with an antibacterial soap, with each sore cleansed carefully. Crusts should be scraped away (soaking them in warm water may ease removal), and an antibiotic ointment should be rubbed into the base of the sore. Some doctors prefer that the child also be given oral antibiotics to prevent complications and hasten healing.

Because impetigo is contagious, special hygienic measures must be observed by each member of the family, with special attention to separating the affected child's towels, bed linens, and clothes for special washing.

If the sores do not stop spreading in three days, or if the child develops an oral temperature over 100°F, parents should consult a doctor for advice. If red streaks or localized swollen glands appear, the child should be taken to his or her doctor. Such signs may mean that the infection is burrowing deeper into tissues, causing an inflammation that may be heralded by redness, swelling, and pain.

Normally, complications do not occur, and parents can be reassured that the unsightly sores of impetigo do not leave permanent scars.

Impulsive behavior

A form of behavior in which the child seems to act without thinking. It is regarded as a major diagnostic feature of an attention deficit disorder.

The child who is impulsive seems unable to wait for anything. Standing in line or waiting a proper turn are impossible tasks. Easily frustrated, the child changes mood quickly and unexpectedly. Adjusting to new routines is quite difficult. In school the impulsive child seems excitable, always making noise or calling out.

Much like the child with HYPERACTIVITY, the impulsive child is generally viewed as unruly and disobedient and is often disciplined. The impulsive child is unable to control his or her need to act and so becomes resistive and angry at the world.

An orderly environment, regularly scheduled breaks and the avoidance of distracting room decorations may help at home. Offering affection when the child is unruly and giving praise when he or she is behaving correctly may also help if parents can be consistent. Appropriate medical and psychological evaluations may point to ways to improve the child's chance for healthy development.

Parents should be careful to remember, however, that until around the age of four, *all* children are impulsive by nature. It's only when the activity is way out of kilter with patterns of most age peers or when the impulsivity carries on into school years and becomes disruptive, that concern is warranted.

Compare HYPERACTIVE BEHAVIOR.

Incest

Strictly speaking, intercourse between two people closely related by blood. Modern descriptions include not only intercourse but any degree of excitation by fondling, and the definition may also be expanded to include stepparents, grandparents, adult caretakers, or other relatives.

Over the past few years there seems to have been a steady increase in media coverage of this serious problem. It remains somewhat unclear whether this mostly reflects lowered barriers about reporting the violation and discussing the subject, or whether there is an actual increase in cases of incest.

Of reported incidents, about 95 percent involve girls between the ages of two and eighteen, most of whom have had their first such experience before age twelve. Three-quarters of the time the offender is either the father or stepfather, and most such involvements last for more than a year. Only 1 percent of incestuous relationships are initiated by adult females. Some authorities believe that sibling incest may be higher even than adult-child contact. It is probable that it is less frequently reported, and, unless there is an extreme difference in age, it seems certain that the experience probably entails a great deal less trauma because it involves two children who probably engage in sex play by mutual consent, rather than an adult-child relationship in which the adult is *always* the responsible party. The myth about little girls being provocative should be relegated to the limbo it deserves. No matter what a young female's behavior, it is the adult who bears responsibility for initiating sex play with a child.

It is not clearly understood why incest, usually between father and daughter, occurs. The families tend to be private and without much outside social interaction. Mother-daughter roles may be reversed in the household. The fathers are often very strict and quite controlling of their daughters' lives. The father may have been exposed to incestuous relationships in his own childhood home. Many times the mothers are sexually remote and, knowingly or unknowingly, contribute to the affair by arranging to be away from home, leaving the father and daughter alone. There is typically little emotional interaction between the mother and the daughter, and the child is not given the strength and self-respect necessary to resist abnormal advances. Overall, there is a distortion of family dynamics that involves all family members. Secrecy becomes of vast importance.

A child or teenager who is being sexually abused may show

signs of EMOTIONAL WITHDRAWAL or DEPRESSION. FEARS and phobias may become pronounced. Nightmares, sleep problems, and regressive behavior such as thumb sucking may be clues. Vague abdominal pain and headaches may signal the emotional stress being suffered.

If it is believed that the child is being molested, a report to a child-abuse agency or protective service is mandatory. What follows—agency intervention, possible severance proceedings, a court order to prevent visitation rights, and so on—may be uncomfortable for all concerned. However, without intervention the consequences are even worse, interfering with the child's normal development and most likely leading to very severe emotional problems that may, in turn, affect the victim's own relationships with future children.

The child or teenager should not be questioned about the specifics of the events any more than is necessary. Support and understanding are crucial, and the girl must be helped to comprehend that this is not her fault and that any future attempt should be reported immediately. Family therapy will most likely be required, and in many cases the child may be removed from the family, at least during a period in which the father is assigned to a counseling group that specializes in the problems of rape and incest.

Indigestion

Imperfect or incomplete digestion, occasionally associated with a disease or some disorder of the digestive system, but most commonly caused by bad eating and drinking habits.

Children should be gently taught to chew their food slowly and thoroughly, and to avoid excitement and strenuous exercise before and immediately after mealtimes.

Eating gas-forming foods such as cabbage or beans or a lot of fried and fatty foods that may be undercooked can also contribute to indigestion. When the child eats the wrong kinds of food or too much food, the stomach and intestines can become distended (overstretched), which interferes with the natural wavelike motions that carry contents through the digestive tract and eliminate waste materials.

Heartburn is one symptom of indigestion. It has nothing

at all to do with the heart but is a burning sensation in the chest caused by some of the stomach's acid contents flowing upward and into the lower part of the esophagus, the delicate lining of which is not designed to deal with acid.

Some relief of simple stomach upset can be obtained by taking one of the many nonprescription antacids. Label instructions for children's doses, if, indeed, the medicine is designed for children to take, should be followed carefully, and it is even better for parents to call a physician for advice. The child should *not* been given aspirin or laxatives, because it is not always possible to be sure the discomfort is only indigestion.

Infantile paralysis

See POLIOMYELITIS.

Infection

The state or condition in which organs or tissues are invaded by pathogenic (disease-causing) organisms. Treatment depends upon the specific organism responsible for the infection.

See also: BACTERIAL INFECTIONS, FUNGUS INFECTIONS, RICKETTSIAL INFECTIONS, VIRAL INFECTIONS, YEAST INFECTIONS.
Compare WORMS.

Infectious mononucleosis

An acute infectious disease caused by the E-B, or Epstein-Barr, virus.

Commonly referred to simply as "mono," it can occur at any age, but it is especially prevalent in young adults, adolescents, and older children, particularly when large groups of young people live in close contact, such as at schools or camps.

The incubation period varies from four to about ten weeks. It is not even quite clear how the infection is transmitted; kissing has often been implicated but is not a major mode of spread.

It starts gradually, and the symptoms are often mild. They are usually sore throat; swollen glands, especially lymph glands in the neck, armpits, and groin; fatigue; and fever. In a few cases a skin rash rather like that of rubella (German measles) develops and, in even rarer cases, the young person may become jaundiced (yellowish). In most cases symptoms subside within a few weeks, although fatigue and malaise (a general sense of being unwell) may persist for several weeks. Sometimes depression and general debility may linger after an unusually severe attack.

Diagnosis is made by a laboratory examination of a blood sample. The disorder causes an increase in certain types of white blood cells called lymphocytes and monocytes, and it may alter their appearance.

No specific treatment is required, although rest may help as long as the young person has a fever. Rough play, contact sports, or any activity which might result in a blow to the abdomen must be avoided. Very often the spleen, an organ in the upper left part of the abdomen, is enlarged and its outer covering tense. In this disease state, the spleen is susceptible to rupture and bleeding, and a surgical emergency may arise.

A return to full activity may be allowed when the child's strength has returned and a doctor's exam has shown that the spleen is not enlarged. Until then, lighter activities may be permitted within the child's fatigue tolerance. The antibiotic ampicillin should not be given because in about 80 percent of mono patients it can cause a skin rash.

Parents need not worry unless serious complications arise. In that case prompt medical attention should be sought. These signs, symptoms, and disorders include CONVULSIONS, ENCEPHALITIS, severe abdominal discomfort that might suggest a ruptured spleen, neck stiffness, pneumonia, and any severe swelling of the tonsils or throat, which could cause serious breathing difficulties.

Influenza

An acute infectious and highly contagious VIRAL INFECTION commonly known as the flu.

Incubation period varies from about twenty-four to about forty-eight hours. Symptoms appear suddenly: severe headache; aches in muscles and joints, especially backache; loss of appetite; sweating; and severe fatigue. Body temperature rises sharply to about 101° to 103°F (38° to 39.5°C). Generally the fever and pain gradually subside within two or three days. Even though high fevers may persist for four or five days in the child with influenza, it's advisable to check with the child's doctor if a temperature over 101° or 102°F has been present for more than twenty-four hours.

In infants and younger children, the signs and symptoms are often similar to those resulting from other viral infections of the respiratory system. Some children will experience FEVER CONVULSION, vomiting, diarrhea, otitis media (middle ear infection), high fever, clear nasal discharge, and fleeting skin rash.

Drugs have no direct effect on the influenza virus, although the antivirus drug amantadine hydrochloride may minimize severity and duration if it is given early on. The latter is only used under very specific circimstances. Other drugs, including antibiotics, may be given to treat a bacterial infection, such as PNEUMONIA.

Otherwise symptomatic treatment is the rule. Activity should be limited until the temperature returns to normal. They should be given plenty of liquids to drink. Light snacks may be offered when the child gets hungry. If the doctor approves, some medication may be given to reduce fever and relieve the pain of headaches. Aspirin should be avoided because of its apparent connection to REYE'S SYNDROME when a child has the flu.

Even when the temperature returns to normal, children often feel weak and slightly dizzy for a few days. A dry, hacking cough may persist for as long as a week or so after the other symptoms have disappeared. However, potentially serious complications from influenza are uncommon in children who are otherwise healthy.

Inner ear infection

See EAR INFECTION.

Insect bites

The bites of many species of insects can cause annoying and sometimes potentially serious symptoms and signs. However, most insect bites require nothing more than a cold compress, the application of cold compresses to the site, or the use of calamine lotion to relieve itching.

An obvious exception to this rule is the relatively uncommon case of ANAPHYLACTIC SHOCK. This reaction may occur in children who are highly sensitive to the bite of a specific insect, and the situation requires immediate, emergency medical attention. Once this condition is known, parents and the child can be provided with certain drugs or treatment kits to keep on hand. Some of the antihistamine drugs can be used to lessen the itching and discomfort.

Children should be strongly discouraged from scratching the place the insect bit; this may worsen the condition. If the bite becomes infected—often signaled by reddening and swelling of the surrounding skin—a doctor should be consulted for appropriate therapy, which may include antibiotics and/or antihistamines more powerful than those that can be obtained without prescriptions.

Compare STINGS.

Insomnia

See SLEEP PROBLEMS.

Intestinal obstruction

An interference with the normal flow of contents through the intestinal tract. It requires immediate medical evaluation and treatment.

Obstructions may be partial or complete, mechanical or metabolic. Strangulated HERNIAS, bands or adhesions, INTUSSUSCEPTION, and congenital (present-at-birth) abnormalities of intestinal formation are the commonest causes in infancy and childhood. Occasionally a newborn baby's bowels will be plugged by too much meconium (a substance created in the baby's intestinal tract while the infant is in the uterus). In rare cases tumors or parasites may be involved, and at times certain infections such as pneumonia or peritonitis may cause an intestinal obstruction.

An infant or child whose intestine is blocked looks very ill. Cramping ABDOMINAL PAIN develops early. Vomiting is usually present and abdominal bloating, a later sign, may be severe. Fevers, respiration that alternates between slow and rapid, and extreme paleness indicate the seriousness of the problem.

If the block is mechanical, it must be relieved, often by surgery. Metabolic or infectious causes must also be medically treated in a vigorous fashion to avoid complications that are a direct threat to life.

See also: PYLORIC STENOSIS.

Intussusception

A form of intestinal obstruction in which one portion of the intestine "telescopes" over another. Although no age group is immune, the condition generally occurs in infants and children under the age of two. It is somewhat more common in boys than in girls.

A child suffers from periods of intense cramping and often screams in pain. The cramping is cyclic in nature, with a period of relief for fifteen or twenty minutes and then a crying out. Sometimes a large, jellylike, bloody bowel movement is passed.

Intussusception is a medical emergency because the blockage impedes blood flow, allowing gangrene to set in. It must be corrected before that happens. Surgery is the most common approach, but a nonsurgical technique involving the rectal introduction of barium may be effective when it alters hydrostatic pressure at the site of intussusception.

Irregular heartbeat

Any deviation from a normal HEART RATE or nature of the beating.

An abnormally fast heartbeat is called tachycardia. It may be associated with hyperthyroidism (an overactive thyroid gland) or some form of heart disease. In paroxysmal tachycardia, the heart suddenly starts to beat rapidly, a fluttering sensation is felt in the chest, and the child may feel faint. Often the episode ends abruptly after just a few minutes. These symptoms can occur in the child with a perfectly healthy heart, but a doctor should be consulted so that a proper diagnosis can be made and treatment can be provided to relieve the distress and anxiety these episodes cause. Sometimes medication is prescribed. Sometimes simple home remedies, such as sucking on crushed ice or lying flat on the floor, are recommended.

An abnormally slow heartbeat is called bradycardia. It may occur in a perfectly healthy child at times, especially in youngsters who are athletes. If not accompanied by faintness or dizziness, it is often considered a healthy sign in the sense of longevity and relative immunity to high blood pressure and other illnesses.

Arrhythmia is the name given to an abnormal rhythm or disturbance of the heartbeat. Some children have a harmless condition known as sinus arrhythmia, in which the PULSE RATE increases when they breathe in and decreases when they breathe out. It is rarely associated with any other symptoms or disease processes.

Compare HEART MURMURS.

Irritability

A reaction in which the infant or child behaves in a testy, petulant, grumpy fashion, frequently crying.

At various times all infants and children become irritable and unhappy. It is only when the behavior tends to be repetitive, frequent, or unusually long-lived that parents need be concerned. Teething is often a cause, as are acute illnesses and fatigue. A milk allergy or other food intolerance may be the cause. If so, diarrhea and unusual or excessive gas will be present. Any EAR INFECTION associated with a cold makes babies cry excessively. An extremely irritable infant with a high fever and vomiting may possibly be developing MENINGITIS. During the newborn period (the first four weeks of life) irritability is a symptom that should never be ignored. Although it might be perfectly benign, the crying could herald the presence of a serious infection. If FEVER or HYPOTHERMIA is present, the need for a medical evaluation is urgent.

Older children usually complain verbally when they are experiencing physical discomfort. Hence, as the child grows, irritability becomes more a signal of emotional stress than it is of a physical problem. Children suffering DEPRESSION are irritable and cry easily. School or peer stresses may make even a healthy child irritable if the pressure builds to significant proportions. Parents can often help by discussing with their children exactly what's bothering them. Reassuring and supportive listening may relieve children by convincing them that their gripes are being taken seriously. Parents should try their very best not to meet irritability with irritability.

If the child's irritability persists, discuss it with the youngster's doctor, who can help sort out possible origins of the problem.

Itching

An irritation of the skin technically known as pruritus that makes one want to scratch the area. It usually results from irritation of pain-registering nerve endings in the skin. With slight stimulation, the nerve ending's response is itching rather than pain. Often the condition is mild and only briefly annoying; sometimes it is so intense and prolonged that normal activities of the child, including sleep, are totally disrupted.

When the cause of itching is associated with a specific infection or disorder, relief occurs from medical treatment of the underlying condition. In other instances the child's doctor may recommend some preparation that can be applied, such as calamine lotion or perhaps a prescription ointment. In many cases severe itching can be relieved by taking a cool bath in water liberally sprinkled with pure baking soda. The child should be discouraged from scratching, which may worsen the condition.

See also: ALLERGY, ANAL ITCHING, CHICKENPOX, DERMATITIS, DIABETES, FUNGUS INFECTION, INSECT BITES, JAUNDICE, JOCK ITCH, KIDNEY DISEASE, LICE, SKIN RASHES, STINGS, VAGINITIS.

J

Jaundice

A yellowish coloring of the skin and often of the whites of the eyes. It is caused when a bile pigment called bilirubin, a breakdown product of the oxygen-carrying part of red blood cells, gets deposited in skin tissues. Jaundice is not a disease but a symptom. Therefore, it is always a signal that medical evaluation is necessary.

Jaundice is present at birth or is observed during the first week of life in approximately 60 percent of full-term babies and about 80 percent of premature infants. This generally occurs because the bilirubin is not broken down, usually because of the immaturity of the liver, or some congenital (present-at-birth) abnormality in the biliary tract. In most cases the symptoms disappear spontaneously, although the nursing and medical staff will be alerted to any underlying disorder, such as a blood group incompatibility, that should be investigated and treated. In older children jaundice is usually a result of liver dysfunction as occurs in hepatitis. When the liver heals the jaundice goes away.

Compare ANEMIA, HEPATITIS.

Jaw pain and swelling

Swelling of the jaw with considerable discomfort is most frequently caused by a dental abscess. The infection may spread deeply into the bone if the situation is untreated.

If causes such as a cut or infected hair follicle are at fault, antibiotics will be needed to clear the infection. SWOLLEN GLANDS may cause a great deal of discomfort, under the jaw. Tumors and cysts of the jaw develop slowly, with swelling and pain being late symptoms.

Caffey's disease, marked by painful jaw swelling and a low-grade fever, may occur in infants. The cause of the disorder is unknown. Symptoms may be present for several months, but no treatment is effective. Eventually the swelling goes down and no deformity remains.

Jealousy

A state or feeling in which the child is resentful of what he or she perceives to be another's good fortune. Adults can understand this better if they stop to remember times that they themselves have felt that someone else is getting more, either materially or emotionally, than they are. Jealousy creates a feeling of anger, usually mild, but at times filled with fairly deep resentment.

It is only when the child almost constantly shows this reaction that parents need be concerned. Often children given to jealousy have serious misgivings about their own worth. They may display irritability and have trouble getting along with peers.

Parents should not reprimand, nor should they remind jealous children of how really fortunate they are. It is best to discuss day-to-day life in a peripheral fashion, looking for clues that might explain why the child may feel put down or left out. Reassure the jealous child frequently, but do it gently and don't make a constant fuss about it. If difficulties persist, talking with the child's doctor or a qualified psychologist may be helpful.

Jock itch

The common name for a FUNGUS INFECTION that causes a scaling, itchy rash in the groin area.

It is rare in children and uncommon in females. However, it can occur in young people, especially adolescent boys. Hot, humid climates and tight-fitting clothing seem to contribute to growth of the fungus, which causes a bright red rash with a very sharp border.

The application of special antifungal solutions or creams will help, as will wearing loose-fitting clothing.

Joint pain

Arthalgia (joint pain) in children is usually caused by some injury. Youngsters are always twisting or turning joints. Mild swelling will usually be present.

Generally speaking, resting the affected part is all that need be involved in treatment. Of course, if there is severe swelling or discoloration and/or the child complains of severe pain, a FRACTURE or a tear of one of the connecting tissues may be present and medical attention should be sought.

Joint pain may also be an early symptom of JUVENILE RHEUMATOID ARTHRITIS, and if fever is present, the joint pain may be signaling RHEUMATIC FEVER.

See also: ANKLE PAIN, HIP PAIN, KNEE PAIN, SHOULDER PAIN.

Juvenile rheumatoid arthritis

Also known as Still's disease, this condition is somewhat similar to rheumatoid arthritis in adults. Typical signs and symptoms include painful and swollen joints (especially larger joints), skin rashes, and swollen lymph glands. A physician may note an enlarged liver and spleen.

Children are often sickest during the development stage of the illness. The body temperature may rise to about 105°F (40°C) and stay that high for several weeks. In some cases there is an associated inflammation of the lungs and the membranes that cover the heart. The child will be lethargic and complain of malaise (a generalized feeling of not being well). In some cases there may be an interference with normal growth and development; this sometimes involves the lower jaw, creating a receding chin line. Juvenile rheumatoid arthritis may occur in early childhood, but rarely before the age of two years. In school-age children it may develop between the ages of eight and twelve. It is more common in girls than in boys, and although the outlook is good compared with adult rheumatoid arthritis, it is a serious and chronic disease that may require physical therapy to help maintain joint mobility and good muscle tone, as well as, in many cases, supportive counseling to help the child and the parents cope with the nature of the disease and the probable need for very long-term therapy.

Treatment is aimed at relieving symptoms and preventing deterioration of the joints. If the latter can be achieved, normal adulthood can be anticipated, since the disease tends to disappear when the child matures. Aspirin or acetaminophen is generally recommended for the relief of symptoms. Occasionally short courses of steroid therapy may be used.

Physical therapy is aimed at preventing permanent deformity or the wasting of muscles. The child and the parents will most likely be taught certain exercises that can be performed at home.

As to emotional impact, the child's doctor or a recommended psychotherapist may be helpful in teaching both the child and the parents how to live with juvenile rheumatoid arthritis.

K

Kidney infections and diseases

Sometimes a BACTERIAL INFECTION will affect a child's kidney tissue or the collecting system that transfers urine to the bladder. Unlike CYSTITIS, kidney infections are frequently associated with high fever and back pain. The child may look quite ill. Abdominal pain and vomiting often make an appearance. The child goes to the bathroom frequently, experiences a burning sensation on urinating, and the urine voided may appear cloudy or bloody.

To avoid long-term kidney damage, these infections must be treated medically. The doctor takes the child's medical history, does a physical examination and lab tests because diagnosis requires certain findings, such as pus in the urine and the growth of bacteria in a culture specimen. Once the acute condition is under control, X rays may be taken and the inside of the bladder may be checked by cystoscopic examination to make sure there is no obstruction to urinary flow, which could cause a backup of pressure against kidney tissue.

Nephritis, the technical term for a kidney inflammation, is not always a result of infection. Sometimes the inflammation seems to start without a known cause, becoming constant and gradually progressing to kidney failure. Some cases are acute and do not become chronic. Some cases are associated with other diseases or seem to have a hereditary basis, or, as in acute glomerulonephritis, may occur because of a previous strep infection.

Once chronic nephritis has severely damaged the kidney, there is nothing that can be done to repair the problem. The child may have to be connected to a dialysis machine several times a week. This machine has tubes that connect with the patient's blood system, so that waste products can be filtered out before the now-purified blood is recirculated.

An alternative method involves surgical transplantation of a normal kidney. This technique requires careful matching and the use of potent medications to minimize the chance of rejection. The operation is effective, sometimes permitting normal functioning over a period of many years. However, side effects can occur, and for many people the cost remains prohibitive.

A disease called nephrosis sometimes occurs in preschool children; it is somewhat more common in boys than in girls. No one is sure what causes it, but it usually starts with a gradual weight gain that reflects edema, the slow but sure accumulation of fluids in the tissues of the body. Although puffiness around the eyes is fairly common early in the disease, the weight gain is often first thought to be normal growth.

Antibiotic and corticosteroid or immunosuppressive drugs are generally prescribed, as well as diuretics (medications that make one urinate more and more frequently) to keep down the excess fluid. Nutritional guidance is usually necessary, as children with nephrosis often lose their appetites. It is especially important for the child to maintain a diet that is low in salt. Also, because infections can cause relapses, parents are generally advised to let the doctor know immediately if the child shows any signs of infection, such as a cough or fever. Finally, some family counseling may be helpful, because children with nephrosis must take special care not to expose themselves to infection, yet they should not be allowed to become loners and should be encouraged to lead as normal a life as possible.

See also: BLOOD IN THE URINE.

Kissing disease

See INFECTIOUS MONONUCLEOSIS.

Knee pain

In children, most discomfort around the knee joint is caused by an injury from a fall or vigorous play. If the blow is a severe one, a FRACTURE or tear in connecting ligaments may be present, especially if there is marked swelling, discoloration, and the child has difficulty moving the knee. When hip pain is present, discomfort in the knee may result from the strain of walking in such a way as to lessen stress at the hip.

Knee pain may be a feature of JUVENILE RHEUMATOID ARTHRITIS and RHEUMATIC FEVER, but then there are other signs and symptoms beyond knee pain. The rapid development of pain, high fever, and swelling may result from an infection. So parents are urged to seek medical evaluation.

A gradually developing swelling and discomfort just below the kneecap is found in Osgood Schlatter's disease. The disorder is caused by a fragmentation of the bone at the upper part of the foreleg, but it is a benign condition that usually responds to rest and the use of aspirin, although in severe cases casting may be necessary.

Knock knees

A posture of the legs in which the knees come together and the lower legs flare outward. During growth at the toddler stage, it is normal for the knees at times to seem too close together. Even if the deformity is marked, it generally corrects itself as the child gets older.

Wedges in shoes do not correct the defect. Only if ligaments around the knee are being stretched is any aggressive therapy, such as bracing, recommended. Even then the knees do not straighten completely; all that happens is that further relaxation of the ligaments is prevented and some correction occurs as the child grows.

On rare occasion rickets or a congenital (present-at-birth) bone disorder may cause abnormalities of the knee joint.

Compare BOWLEGS.

L

Laryngitis

Inflammation of the larynx (the voice box). An acute attack can develop suddenly because of overusing the voice, as in shouting, cheering, singing, or otherwise abusing the vocal cords. Laryngitis may also develop from an upper respiratory viral infection like the common cold, bronchitis, tonsillitis, sore throat, sinusitis, pertussis (whooping cough), or measles.

Symptoms include hoarseness, a tickling sensation or pain in the throat, difficulty in swallowing, and, if the larynx is swollen, shortness of breath on physical exertion or other BREATHING DIFFICULTIES.

Chronic laryngitis can result from inadequate treatment of repeated acute attacks or from starting to overuse the voice again before the larynx has fully healed. Swollen tissues may become thickened with scar tissue, leading to permanent damage to the voice. Irritants, including smoke, can lead to further thickening of the vocal cords and cartilage tissues of the larynx.

Laryngitis can be an early sign of CROUP. If severe, croup demands a doctor's careful examination. Sometimes antibiotics are prescribed to treat any associated bacterial infection.

Lazy eye

See STRABISMUS.

Learning disability

A broad term to describe a performance that falls short of expectations for the child's peers in age, and which cannot be accounted for by lack of schooling.

A correctable impairment can result from a HEARING LOSS or a visual disorder such as FARSIGHTEDNESS or NEARSIGHTEDNESS. However, MENTAL RETARDATION, DYSLEXIA, and ATTENTION DEFICIT DISORDERS may be responsible. Parents should see that the child with an apparent learning disability gets an especially thorough physical examination before he or she is tested for neurologic or emotional problems.

Leg cramps

Children most often suffer leg cramps because of excessive running, climbing, and general horseplay. After a few minutes the pain goes away, and they are off and running again.

Sometimes a day's activities will cause later cramping, so that the child awakens during the night, crying or complaining. A warm bath, a children's dose of an aspirinlike medication, and massaging the legs will often relieve the pain. Symptoms may persist over several days or weeks, but the problem eventually goes away by itself as the child's leg muscles strengthen.

Leg cramping and other muscular cramps may plague teenage athletes at times of extreme exertion. Plenty of liquids should be taken to replace the loss of body fluids and the imbalance of salts that cause the discomfort.

On rare occasions improper footwear may cause muscles to tire too quickly so that a child or adolescent suffers leg pain or cramping.

Leukemia

A form of cancer in which there is an abnormal, uncontrolled multiplication of immature leukocytes (white blood cells). These cells cannot function normally, and they also eventually infiltrate other tissues, such as bone marrow, preventing the production of the other components of normal blood. The failure of red cell formation leads to anemia; the immaturity of the white cells lowers the body's resistance to infection; and the lack of platelet production increases the risk of abnormal bleeding. Therefore anemia, infection, and bleeding are common signs.

Fairly early on the child with acute lymphatic leukemia will show increased fatigue, a pale complexion, unexplained fever, repeated infections, and an abnormal amount of bruising that cannot be accounted for. The examining physician will probably note an enlarged liver or spleen. Laboratory findings generally include a large increase, or at times a decrease, in white blood cells, many of which are immature, and lowered red cell and platelet counts. The confirming diagnosis is made by examining a specimen of bone marrow.

The acute lymphatic type of leukemia accounts for about 80 percent of all childhood cases. Current treatment, such as chemotherapy, transfusions, and antibiotics to fight associated bacterial infection, allows about 90 percent of the children to enjoy a period of remission, in which symptoms temporarily go away, and about 50 percent survive longer than five years after diagnosis.

There are several forms of the disease, such as acute lymphocytic leukemia, and acute granulocytic leukemia (AGL), which is much more common in adults. Therapeutic results vary, although some period of remission is usually achieved.

Since leukemia is potentially a fatal disease, the parents, the child, and any siblings may benefit greatly from counseling that helps them understand the disease's impact and how they can participate most actively in the course of treatment.

Lice

Infestation with lice, a condition known as pediculosis, is far more common than the general public tends to think. Although it most often is a problem when a child's hair, skin, and clothing are not kept clean, children can and do inadvertently acquire lice by coming into contact with infested people or articles, for example, a comb, a hat, or someone else's jacket. Most schools report at least one outbreak of lice during each school term, so parents should not be ashamed or feel that their household is dirty if children become infested.

First signs are usually intense itching, irritation, and inflammation or redness of the skin. Lice are frequently found on the scalp and in the hair, but also on the body, especially on hairy parts. The eggs or nits have small grayish bodies, stick to the hair and cannot be brushed off; they take about two weeks to hatch. The eggs of body lice tend to be laid in clothing and underclothing, especially along seams. Body lice cause itching across the abdomen and back and sometimes produce hivelike rashes. Pubic lice affect not only the pubic area but also the thighs and lower abdomen.

Treatment of lice on the eyelashes can be started by applying a Vaseline-like product to the eyelid margins for a few days and then removing the nits.

Probably the first rule of treatment is to avoid scratching, which can cause a bacterial infection. The hair should be thoroughly lathered with a special shampoo, then rinsed and dried. Dip a fine-toothed comb into vinegar and run it through the hair repeatedly from the scalp outward. Nits can also be removed one by one with the fingers or tweezers if parents are patient and take their time.

Although some lice medications are available without a prescription, it is best to ask the child's doctor for a recommendation. A shampoo or lotion containing 1 percent gamma benzene hydrochloride, available by prescription, is often effective when used as the doctor instructs. Children may return to school after the first treatment. The current recommendation is that the child should be retreated a week after the first application.

If one child is infested, everyone in the family should be carefully inspected and treated if necessary. The child's clothing, towels, bedding, hairbrushes, combs, barrettes, curlers, and head gear should be boiled. If an item can't be boiled, it should be washed in the hottest water possible and then ironed. Dry cleaning is also effective.

Lightheadedness

See DIZZINESS.

Limping

Any unusual manner of walking through which the child tries to limit movement of the hip, knee, or ankle.

If this situation persists for more than a couple of days, even if connected to an obvious injury, the child should be evaluated by a physician. The limping may reflect a problem in the joint being favored, but in some cases it may be caused by a tumor or injury of the bone shaft or muscle or by an orthopedic problem that requires treatment.

Importantly, any child who is limping and has a fever should be seen by a doctor immediately.

Liver disorders

The liver is a large organ located in the upper right-hand side of the abdominal cavity. It serves many important functions; the body cannot survive without it. It manufactures bile and bile salts necessary for digestion. It also manufactures and stores materials needed for the process of blood coagulation. It stores sugar required for energy. It also detoxifies the body by removing waste products from the bloodstream and breaking them down so they can be eliminated. In short, metabolism is its primary function.

Liver structure is relatively immature in infants, especially premature babies, so certain metabolic deficiencies may occur and jaundice will temporarily be present. In a condition known as galactosemia, abnormal metabolism of carbohydrates may cause childhood cirrhosis of the liver, accompanied by mental retardation. HEPATITIS is generally accompanied by abdominal pain and vomiting and may develop as a feature of INFECTIOUS MONONUCELOSIS. Occasionally tumors and cysts develop within liver tissue.

Lockjaw

See TETANUS.

Low blood sugar

See HYPOGLYCEMIA.

Lupus erythematosus

A chronic disease of unknown origin, which is both systemic (affecting large portions of the body) and cutaneous (affecting the skin). It is considered a collagen disease (collagen is the supportive material that holds skin, tendons, bones, cartilage, and connective tissue together). Some authorities believe that it is an autoimmune disease, that is, one in which the body's natural defense system malfunctions and produces antibodies against some of the sufferer's own tissue.

The disease is not common in children, but when it does

occur it is usually more acute and more serious than in adults. Early symptoms include fever, pain and inflammation of the joints, and skin rash. In some cases a red patch forms on the face and over the bridge of the nose (the so-called butterfly rash). The skin eruptions may spread to the neck, chest, and extremities, although only about one-third of the children with lupus will experience this effect, which is worsened by exposure to sunlight. Many children experience malaise (a general feeling of being unwell), loss of appetite, and loss of weight.

Systemic lupus erythematosus, also known as disseminated lupus, is a progressive and potentially fatal disease that can affect the functioning of the lungs, kidneys, and heart. Treatment depends on the severity of the disease and which organs are affected. A particularly dangerous complication in children is the development of nephritis (inflammation of the kidneys). Corticosteroids are generally prescribed. Modern treatment methods allow more than 85 percent of lupus-stricken children to survive for at least 10 years, and some may escape the fatal outcome that was once prevalent.

Milder forms of the disease have an even more favorable outlook. Topical steroid preparations can be used for facial rash, and other drugs are prescribed to relieve pain and inflammation of affected joints. Antimalarial drugs such as hydroxychloroquine are sometimes useful. The main goal is to relieve symptoms and to control or suppress any associated disease of the kidneys or other internal organs.

Lying

If the child is younger than four, be cautious about calling his or her untruth a lie. Young children normally have some trouble distinguishing between reality and fantasy, so a tall tale about a horse walking down the sidewalk may not be a real *lie.*

Healthy older children may tell a few lies now and then, often as a means of escaping punishment for some wrongdoing. On occasion children may lie in an effort to seem more powerful or stronger than they are.

Only when parents see a pattern of lying develop should they be concerned. Sometimes children latch on to lying to get other children or adults to do what they want them to do. This is manipulative behavior and could spell future psychological trouble for the child.

Punishment does not work unless parents are absolutely certain the child has lied. Also, the punishment should fit the crime. Screaming and physically striking children only brings more denials and an increased motivation for lying to escape such punishment. With patience, parents can teach children that lying is neither acceptable nor profitable. They have to be helped to understand the consequences of misbehavior, and exactly how they will be disciplined. For a time, more supervision may be in order so lies can be nipped in the bud.

Lymphangitis

Inflammation of lymphatic channels or vessels.

As the lymphatic system tries to remove or drain off infection, lymph channels become inflamed, creating thick, red lines. Occasionally the lymph glands that drain an area of infection become swollen and tender.

In rare instances the original site of infection may need to be drained surgically. Usually antibiotics will cure the infection and the red streaks will disappear.

See also: SWOLLEN GLANDS.

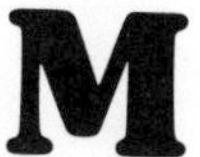

M

Malabsorption syndrome

Any of a variety of conditions that affect the intestines or digestive glands in such a way that causes some failure in absorption of one or more nutrients essential for health.

The most common sign, called steatorrhea, is the passing of loose stools that contain excessive fat. The stools are pale, bulky, and so light that they may require several flushes for complete toilet disposal. Other signs and symptoms include weight loss, abdominal bloating, muscle wasting, anorexia (diminished appetite), and audible gurgling or splashing sounds coming from the intestine.

A specific although fairly uncommon example of a malabsorption disorder is called celiac disease or nontropical sprue. It tends to run in families, and the child may be affected as young as six months. If it is untreated, celiac disease of childhood is typified by abdominal bloating, steatorrhea, muscle wasting, loss of appetite, severe diarrhea, stunted growth, and general listlessness.

In celiac disease the digestive tract cannot tolerate gluten, a component of wheat and other cereals. In some way not yet understood, gluten damages the lining of the intestines in those who are sensitive to the substance. The treatment is simple: avoid gluten; the results are dramatically good. However, avoiding gluten may not be easy because, in addition to the more obvious foods such as wheat flour and cereals, it may be present in cakes, cookies, and bread. The child's doctor can provide parents with a list of foods and recipes that are gluten free.

Because malabsorption syndromes occur with different frequencies at different ages (some may be discovered shortly after birth) and because treatment is based on the specific underlying cause, parents are urged to seek medical evaluation of any child who seems to be showing signs of malnourishment and/or marked gastrointestinal upset.

Malignancy

Growing worse; posing a direct threat to life; harmful. The term is frequently used as a synonym for a cancerous growth.

See also: CANCER.

Mastitis

See BREASTS.

Mastoiditis

Inflammation of any part of the mastoid—that prominent piece of spongy bone just behind the earlobe. Its air cavities lead directly to the middle ear, so middle-ear infections sometimes spread to the mastoid process.

An early symptom is intense pain behind the ear. The child's temperature may rise slightly, the pulse rate may become rapid, there may be a discharge from the affected ear, and hearing loss will be fairly pronounced. If an abscess develops within the mastoid's air cells, swelling behind the ear can be quite noticeable.

Before the days of antibiotic therapy, mastoiditis often meant surgical removal of a section of bone so that pus could be drained. Today the early diagnosis and treatment of EAR INFECTION means that the mastoid is less frequently affected. Even when it is, antibiotic therapy, generally continued over a period of two weeks, is quite effective. Only in advanced cases in which the child has not received appropriate medical treatment might there be a need for surgical drainage.

As with any ear problem, the child should be taken to a doctor as soon as the slightest indication of mastoiditis appears. This will reduce the risk of further complications, including possible MENINGITIS.

Masturbation

Self-manipulation of one's genitals for sexual excitation or gratification.

Self-exploration is part of children's normal curiosity about their own bodies. Once they find that handling their genitals is pleasurable, they then masturbate because it feels good. This behavior is normal; it may even enhance their sex lives once they become adults.

Parents should not express concern, nor should they try to shame children or frighten them by telling myths about a part falling off, or hair growing on one's hands, or other falsehoods that were often related in more repressive eras. Properly approached, masturbation becomes just a small part of a child's overall experience and no difficulties arise from it.

However, compulsive masturbation is often a means of releasing tensions accumulating because of an emotional problem, marital tension in the child's family, undue sibling rivalry, or a feeling of rejection by peers or family members. In children who are affected, masturbation may occur with extreme frequency, conspicuously, and at inappropriate times and places. If the parents become upset and punitive, the situation seems to worsen. Hence evaluation by a professional is advised.

MBD

See ATTENTION DEFICIT DISORDERS.

Measles

A highly contagious VIRAL INFECTION with a typical red skin rash and grain-sized white spots on a red base, called Koplik's spots, in the mouth. The incubation period is from about ten to fourteen days. First signs are fever, runny nose, red and watery eyes, sneezing, and a hacking cough. The temperature generally continues to rise slightly every day for about three or four days and may go as high as 104°F (40°C). It is about this time that the Koplik's spots may sometimes be seen on the inner surface of the cheeks; the spots appear and disappear rapidly, usually within twelve to eighteen hours.

The rash begins behind the ears and spreads to the face and neck. Within the next day or two it spreads to the body and limbs, becomes blotchy in places, increases in size, and changes to a slightly darker color.

The eyes of children with measles are especially sensitive to light for the first few days. It is not necessary to darken the room, but strong lights should be avoided. If the child's eyelids tend to stick together, the doctor may prescribe some special eyedrops. When the fever is high, cool sponging offers some relief, and the child should be offered tempting liquids frequently. Sometimes a mechanical moisturizer is useful.

Aside from relieving symptoms, there is little treatment for measles—other than prevention by prior immunization. Because it is caused by a virus, it will not respond to antibiotics.

Most cases of measles present no serious problems, but the doctor will want to make sure that there is not also an infection of the eyes, ears, or lungs. In very rare instances bleeding from the mouth, nose, or bowels (hemorrhagic measles) may develop. Parents should immediately call the child's doctor if this happens.

Compare RUBELLA, CHICKENPOX.

Meckel's diverticulum

A small outpouching of the intestinal wall, at the far end of the small intestine. The defect occurs when a duct normally present before birth fails to disappear altogether.

A Meckel's diverticulum may cause problems if the tissue becomes irritated and bleeds or perforates. Its presence is often determined only after a search for the cause of anemia is made.

Bleeding may be slow and scant in amount, and rarely is it associated with pain. When it does occur, abdominal pain is vague and centers around the navel. On some occasions a Meckel's diverticulum may cause an intestinal obstruction, and if the inflammation is severe or a perforation is present, the child may show symptoms resembling those of acute appendicitis.

Meningitis

Inflammation of the meninges, the three delicate membranes that cover the brain. It is generally caused by bacterial or viral microorganisms.

The infection often spreads to the meninges from other sites such as the ears, sinuses, tonsils, or upper respiratory tract. This spread is not a direct one, but rather one in which the organisms are carried up the bloodstream. The first symptoms are common to many other infections: high temperature, chills, severe headache, and vomiting. Lethargy and irritability are common. Marked stiffness of the neck is a prominent sign; the child's head may bend back and he or she cannot bend it forward. Infants may show a bulging fontanel or soft spot, and as pressure within the skull increases, they may cry out in a shrill, high-pitched tone. Convulsions may occur, as well as coma. Children with meningitis may also be in a state of blood-system shock if the bacteria get into the bloodstream. A purplish rash, caused by widespread blockage of small blood vessels, may occur.

Immediate medical attention is required for this serious condition. Hospitalization is the rule, and the medical team will most likely do a spinal tap, that is, take a sample of cerebrospinal fluid (fluid in the spinal canal) to confirm the diagnosis. It will be analyzed not only for specific organisms but also for the prevalence of certain white blood cells, protein content, sugar content, and other diagnostic signs.

Antibiotic treatment is used. With prompt and proper treatment, the chances of complete and uncomplicated recovery from meningitis are very good.

Compare ENCEPHALITIS.

Menstrual difficulties

Disorders of menstruation, such as delayed onset, abnormal bleeding, and excessive pain, are not uncommon in adolescents. Extremely complex hormonal and anatomical processes are involved, and it normally takes some time for these systems to function smoothly and regularly.

Parents should be sure that their daughters know about menstruation before it occurs. A good time may be when the girl first starts to show physical signs of sexual development (breast buds), although younger children may express interest in the subject. Several pamphlets and books are available that explain the process in understandable language. But nothing is quite so comforting as a personal talk, in which the normality of menstrual bleeding can be stressed and the girl may be encouraged to regard this as a sign of growing maturity rather than a nuisance. Most frequently the girl will prefer to talk with her mother or another female caretaker, since pubescent children are often embarrassed about sex and may feel more comfortable talking with a woman they know well.

Cramping abdominal discomfort, backache, and leg aches are common complaints. Tension aggravates these symptoms, and severe anxiety about menstruation may result in vomiting, paleness, and occasional fainting. If school attendance or other activities are interrupted, medications are available, but it is advisable that the girl consult with her doctor so that the situation can be evaluated and the prescription will be one appropriate for a teenager.

Parents should be reassured that it may take several months for a regular menstrual pattern to become established. Bleeding may be spotty one time and normal the next. Sometimes as long as six months may elapse between periods. Excessive or prolonged flow (lasting more than a week) should be reported to the girl's doctor.

Most girls in the United States start their periods at around twelve years of age. Only if the delay goes beyond sixteen need a doctor be consulted, unless other symptoms are present.

Far more often than not, teenagers' menstrual difficulties clear up of their own accord. However, if discomfort remains severe, irregularity continues, bleeding is heavy and prolonged, or there is an excessive delay in menarche (onset of menstruation), the young girl should definitely see her doctor. Possible causes of abnormal menstrual difficulties include conditions that affect the hypothalamus or the thyroid gland, nutritional deficits, emotional stress, chromosomal and endocrine disorders, as well as the use of certain drugs that may have been prescribed for other conditions.

Mental retardation

Delayed development in language, social, and adaptive skills so that the child fails to reach the level of functioning appropriate for his or her age. Causes of mental retardation are varied: genetic factors, usually with a family history of prior mental retardation; chromosomal and metabolic abnormalities; prenatal or at-birth infections; maternal drug abuse; injuries; and so on. However, medical experts estimate that in approximately 80 percent of cases, the cause cannot be determined.

Parents of a mentally retarded child should know their child's category of retardation so they can have some input into determining the most appropriate learning environment and how best to structure the home environment if the child is to continue living with the family.

Psychological evaluation is essential. According to the child's age, the most popular tests, listed from under two to fifteen years and eleven months, are the Bayley Scale of Infant Development, the Stanford-Binet, the Wechsler Preschool and Primary Scale of Intelligence, and the Wechsler Intelligence Scale for Children. For children up to five years, the Denver Developmental Screening Test provides some approximation of intelligence level. The categories of retardation are:

Borderline children (IQ 84 to 71) have trouble learning in a regular school. But once out of school, they tend to blend into the general population. They can support themselves at jobs that are not too demanding. Approximately 14 percent of all children tested in schools are in this group.

Mildly retarded children (IQ 70 to 50) are termed educable. Some of them can be taught to read up to a fourth- to sixth-grade level, and so many of them, too, can be expected to be self-supporting in menial jobs.

Moderately retarded children (IQ 49 to 35) are termed trainable. That is, they can generally be expected to take care of their personal needs of dressing, washing, eating, and the like, and they may gather some minimal social skills. But they generally always require a structured, supportive environment. Partly because of obvious language and motor impairments, and partly because their thinking is so concrete and very-young-childlike, they are apt to experience considerable trouble dealing with the outside world.

Severely retarded children (IQ 34 to 20) are somewhat trainable, but to a *far* lesser degree than the moderately retarded child. Therefore, they require a highly supervised, structured environment.

Profoundly retarded children (IQ 19 and below) usually cannot even learn to walk, let alone talk. Vocalizations are usually confined to unintelligible grunts, and it is totally unreasonable to expect such a child to attain any degree of self sufficiency.

Parents should also be aware of the fact that, just as may happen with children who have normal intelligence or higher, mental illness can occur in the mentally retarded. It may be harder to diagnose and treat because of the child's limited verbal skills. However, it may manifest itself in many ways, including destructive behavior disorders.

Once the degree of retardation is established, the child's parents, and any siblings, should consult with appropriate specialists who can assist them in making decisions about the child's home setting, educational programs, and the setting of realistic goals for everyone involved. Genetic counseling may also be useful if the mental retardation is thought or known to be familial.

Milk allergy

Some children are allergic (particularly sensitive) to one or more of the proteins in cow's milk. The disorder is sometimes called cow's milk protein sensitivity.

In infants from birth to about six months, typical signs and symptoms are fever, vomiting, diarrhea (with watery stools sometimes tinged with blood), steatorrhea (excessive amounts of fat in bowel movements), weight loss or failure to gain weight, and anemia. Some babies may develop severe and persistent diarrhea that directly interferes with the absorption of essential nutrients by the small intestines. In rare cases the infant may even experience anaphylactic shock.

A second basic form of milk allergy is usually first noted when the hypersensitive child is between the ages of six months and two years. Signs and symptoms may include wheezing, nasal congestion, swelling, constant or intermittent diarrhea, and a failure to thrive resulting from the digestive tract's failure to absorb nutrient proteins properly.

Once the diagnosis is made, cow's milk must be eliminated from the child's diet for a period of time. It can be replaced with a special hypoallergenic formula. If the symptoms disappear and then the child once again reacts badly to cow's milk, the diagnosis is confirmed and the youngster is placed back on the hypoallergenic formula.

For reasons not clearly understood, many of these children are able to tolerate cow's milk once they grow older. Most pediatricians recommend that children be kept on the hypoallergenic formula for at least one year before cow's milk is reintroduced into their diets.

See also: ALLERGY.

Milk intolerance

This disorder differs from a MILK ALLERGY. It occurs because of an inability to digest lactose (milk sugar) and may have a hereditary basis.

Some infants will develop this intolerance after having a viral gastroenteritis. Whatever the cause, some infants and children experience abdominal discomfort, gassiness, and diarrhea when given milk. A few weeks on a soybean milk formula gives the intestine time to heal, and the problem should clear up. Children who continue to suffer discomfort or diarrhea after they have drunk milk should be given substitute products as recommended by a doctor.

Minimal brain dysfunction

See ATTENTION DEFICIT DISORDERS.

Mole

See BIRTHMARK.

Mongolism

See DOWN'S SYNDROME.

Moniliasis

See THRUSH, YEAST INFECTION.

Mononucleosis

See INFECTIOUS MONONUCLEOSIS.

Moodiness

A form of behavior in which children or adolescents generally become quiet and avoid interacting with people around them. Depending on various factors behind this behavior, the withdrawal may last a day or two, with an abrupt return to normal. At times mood swings, from very sad to very joyful, may be quite wide.

Adolescents are especially given to wide mood swings. From an adult's viewpoint, these periods of moodiness may seem inappropriate in the context of what is really happening. A sixteen-year-old may be bouncy and cheerful as he leaves for school, even though rain is pouring down, his best friend just moved away, and he failed an important examination. The next day may be bright and sunny, his best friend calls to invite him for a long weekend, and he gets an A in an even more important examination, but he snaps at everyone all during dinner and then retires to his room to listen to his stereo and stare off into space.

It is not as important to understand such behavior as it is to *accept* it as normal.

Preadolescents generally tend to be much less moody; if moodiness does occur, it will most likely be a reaction to stress at school, with peers, or other family members, and it does not last long.

Of course, if the child or adolescent seems to have unusually long or severe bouts of moodiness, or when symptoms of DEPRESSION seem to be present and parents can't seem to discover a source or a solution in a supportive, nonconfrontative discussion, it may be wise to seek professional help.

Motion sickness

Many children are susceptible to motion sickness, sometimes called travel sickness, which is caused by the effects of irregular or rhythmic movements as they cause two small motion detectors in the inner ear to do "flip-flops." Nausea, dizziness, and even vomiting may occur.

Often children outgrow this tendency. Until they do, parents can ensure more comfortable trips by administering children's doses of nonprescription antihistamine products such as Antivert, Bonine, Dramamine, Emetrol, Marezine, Tigan, Trave-Arex, or Vertrol. As with any medication, it is essential that label instructions be followed to the letter and that very young children not be given some medications. When in doubt, call the child's doctor for advice.

Motor development

The child's growing capacity to perform certain movements and tasks.

There is a great deal of variation within the age ranges at which children develop certain motor skills. Nonetheless, some general expectations may be helpful to parents:

Age	Activity
at birth	Grasp reflex (able to hold the parent's finger, etc.)
3–4 months	Sits if supported
4–5 months	Can reach intentionally
7–8 months	Sits alone
6–10 months	Grasps with palm, grasps with thumb and forefinger
12–13 months	Stands alone briefly
12–15 months	Walks briefly without assistance
2 years	Climbs on furniture, walks up stairs one at a time, can build six-block tower
3 years	Can ride tricycle, can build three-block bridge, can make a cross with a crayon
3–6 years	Adds many more skills, like skating or jumping rope, as muscles strengthen and speed increases
7 years	Can bathe self, use a crayon to copy a drawing of a diamond, can tie a bow knot
8 years	Can use table knife
9 years	Bathes without assistance

If parents have any question about their child's motor development, they should check with a doctor. Many factors are involved, and parents should not worry unduly if their child seems to fall behind other children slightly.

Mouth-to-mouth resuscitation

See CARDIOPULMONARY RESUSCITATION.

Mumps

A VIRAL INFECTION of the salivary glands located along the jaw that especially affects the parotid gland, located just in front of the ear. The virus can be spread through the breath of the infected child, who may then transmit the disease within forty-eight hours even though he or she won't come down with the disease until the incubation period of two or three weeks has passed. Because of its long incubation period, mumps spreads throughout a family or a school long before individual sufferers show signs of the disease.

Children between the ages of five and fifteen are most susceptible, although it is possible to catch mumps at any age. One bout of mumps normally provides protection for life; there is also an immunization shot that should be given to anyone over the age of fifteen months.

First signs are stiffness and slight pain in the neck, followed by a swelling of the parotid gland, which greatly enlarges the entire side of the neck and cheek, usually on one side but sometimes on both. A child may have difficulty opening the mouth, the mouth may become quite dry, and fever is present. In severe cases there may be vomiting, and the temperature can go as high as 104°F (40°C).

Most cases of mumps are relatively mild, discounting the neck discomfort, and the swelling usually recedes in five to ten days. There is no special therapy other than keeping the mouth clean and refreshed with gargles or mouth washes and offering plenty of liquids. Some children will feel some relief of discomfort if a hot water bottle is placed along the neck; others will prefer an ice pack. Parents can apply whichever feels better to the child.

Complications are rare in younger children, but adolescents may sometimes get an infection of the pancreas, thyroid gland, testicles, or ovaries. When complications do occur in childhood, they may be in the form of ENCEPHALITIS (an inflammation of the brain). However, this occurs in only about 250 out of 100,000 cases and carries a mortality rate of only about 2 percent.

Murmurs

See HEART MURMURS.

Muscular dystrophy

A group of disorders characterized by gradual and progressive degeneration (wasting away) of muscle fibers; it eventually causes crippling, and children may be fitted with leg braces only to find themselves having to use a wheelchair soon afterward.

The exact origin of muscular dystrophy is not clear, but at least half of those children suffering from the disease have a family history in which at least one member of the direct family line, of either sex, is affected. It is thought to be associated with an inherited difficulty in the ability of muscles to take up amino acid (a protein) and use it for normal metabolic activities. This probably occurs because of an enzyme deficiency. The result is atrophy (muscle wasting) instead of growth. Classification depends on age of onset, the rate at which weakness progresses, and how the muscular involvement is distributed throughout the body.

Boys are affected more often than girls. Sometimes the youngster will waddle like a duck, have trouble climbing stairs, and fall frequently. The muscles of the chest, abdomen, and buttocks are affected first; then the disease progresses steadily to involve other body parts. As a general rule, disability is fastest in children in whom the disease appears early in life, say, at or before the age of three. Most children with muscular dystrophy are confined to a wheelchair by the time they are ten or twelve.

There is no cure and no specific treatment for this group of diseases. Strenuous exercise should be avoided because it can hasten the breakdown of muscle fibers. On the other hand, children should be kept moderately active and walking for as long a time as possible, both for psychological reasons and to minimize muscle contractures and deformities. To keep the child functioning fairly normally for as long as possible, it will be necessary to enlist the aid of many people, including, for example, school personnel, who may be able to help arrange for transportation and see to special needs such as toilet facilities the child can use. Diet should be low in calories, to help prevent too much weight gain. All infections should be treated promptly, especially upper respiratory infections, since the child with muscular dystrophy develops difficulty in expanding the chest and/or coughing. Counseling with experts in the field may be useful to the entire family, for muscular dystrophy afflicts not only the affected child but everyone who is close to the child.

Muscle cramps

See LEG CRAMPS.

Muscle pain

Muscular discomfort, technically called myalgia, frequently occurs in children simply because of strenuous physical exertion. When muscles are stressed, there is some tissue swelling and an accumulation of metabolic waste products. With rest, the muscle fibers return to their normal state.

Certain viral infections may cause muscle pain. Influenza illnesses sometimes induce varying degrees of muscle discomfort that may last for some time after other symptoms are gone. Rest and the use of children's doses of aspirinlike drugs offer some relief until healing occurs.

JUVENILE RHEUMATOID ARTHRITIS and other connective-tissue diseases cause muscle pain along with joint swelling and fevers or skin rashes. On rare occasion tumors of muscle tissue itself cause discomfort confined to a particular area.

Muscles may also be strained by improperly fitted shoes or by orthopedic problems in the legs. Two rather rare diseases may cause muscle pain, too. One is trichinosis, a parasitic infection usually acquired by eating undercooked pork. Polymyositis is an inflammatory muscle-tissue disorder for which no cause is known; large muscle groups are affected, and the pain is associated with weakness. The neck muscles may be affected first, and children have difficulty lifting their heads. Cortisone treatment brings good results, although the problem may recur later in life.

Muscle weakness

The progressive loss of strength and normal function of a muscle or muscle group.

Some families have a rare genetic disorder in which periodic episodes of weakness occur. This disorder, called familial periodic paralysis, was formerly considered essentially untreatable, aside from resting after an attack. Currently doctors prescribe oral potassium chloride and acetazolamide for control of symptoms.

MUSCULAR DYSTROPHY is a disease in which muscle weakness is the predominant feature. An untreated THYROID DISORDER, either hyper- or hypothyrodism, can also cause muscle weakness.

Because muscle weakness, sometimes accompanied by muscle pain, may indicate a serious disorder, parents are advised to arrange for their child's medical evaluation whenever any signs of weakness, such as difficulty climbing stairs, getting up from a sitting position, or an unusual manner of walking, is noticed.

Myopia

See NEARSIGHTEDNESS.

N

Nail biting

Biting is considered by most mental health authorities to be a sign of aggression. Often very young children bite their own nails in an effort to control acts of aggression they may not want to direct outward. Nail biting may also offer a child something to do when the environment is not very stimulating or when he or she would rather be screaming but subconsciously senses that chewing is the wiser choice. Whatever the origin(s), nail biting eventually becomes a habit.

Parents should not scold or punish the child. Many children will outgrow the habit when they learn to care about their own appearance. Also, if it is done in private and is not so extensive as to resemble anything more than very close clipping, it may be best to ignore the situation.

However, if the nail biting is severe enough to prohibit normal nail growth, causes small skin breaks that can become infected, or the child nail bites compulsively, then some steps should be taken.

On occasion the unraveling of some stressful problem enables the child to stop nail biting. More often than not a direct behavioral therapy approach works best. Try establishing a schedule in which the child may chew all the nails *except* the pinkies for a period of two weeks, at which time some definite, preset reward will be given. Next, the child may bite all the nails except the pinkies and the ring fingers, again with a reward in mind. Repeat this until all the fingers have been eliminated as chewable. During all this time a substitute chewable such as sugarless gum or mints might be offered.

Parents should be patient. The biting became a habit slowly; so will the nonbiting. Only if severe nail biting is accompanied by other signs of undue stress, such as emotional withdrawal or very easily aroused anger, need professional advice be sought.

Nails

For the first several months of life, babies' nails are soft and pliable, often splitting before attaining much length. If cutting is needed, parents should be careful not to cut too close to the fingertips. Rounding with a soft emery board is even better, since if clipping should accidentally break the skin, an easy route for infection exists. Toenails should be cut straight across and with enough length left so that nail margins extend slightly beyond the soft tissues of the toe. This method will avoid ingrown toenails, especially as the child begins to walk and wear shoes.

Some teenage girls complain of fingernail splitting, which is caused by brittleness. Although there may be some underlying abnormality of nail structure, the problem is aggravated by filing, by using nail-polish removers, and by too frequent contact with soap and water. Treatment includes applying hand creams around the nail bed, gentle manicuring, and, if the girl chooses, several layers of polish to discourage splitting.

Paronychia (infections around the nail bed) may occur and must be treated by a physician. Antibiotics are prescribed, and if soaking according to the doctor's suggestion does not allow for proper draining, surgical drainage may have to be done.

Injury to nails may cause a whitish discoloration or a collection of blood beneath the affected nail. The pain may be extremely intense, even though the injury cannot be classified as dangerous. Again, medical help should be sought; the doctor may shave the nail or release the pressure by applying heated metal.

When an injury causes loss of a nail, parents, and the child, need to be patient. It will take a fingernail some three to six months and a toenail some six to eight months to grow back.

Nails also serve as a clue to general health. Bluish nails may signal some heart or blood-vascular disorder. Pale nails may be present in anemia. Nutritional deficits may also be signaled by discoloration of the nails, and certain deformities, such as ridges or pitting, may indicate other generalized disease, sometimes of a congenital (present-at-birth) nature. If parents note any of these abnormalities, they should speak with a doctor and arrange for the child's medical examination.

Nasal congestion

The common cold is responsible for nasal congestion more than all other causes combined. Children can be expected to have as many as thirty such viral infections before they reach the age of ten.

Decongestants may be helpful, although many authorities question how effective these drugs are, and many doctors warn against the frequent use of decongestant nasal sprays because they can cause a rebound effect, that is, the congestion will reappear in an even more severe form. Vaporizer and saltwater sprays or drops seem to be the most effective means of relieving the discomfort of nasal congestion. In infants, suctioning with a nasal bulb syringe after giving nose drops will allow easier feeding and better sleep.

An ALLERGY can frequently cause prolonged periods of severe nasal congestion. If symptoms limit the child's activity, consult a doctor about the advisability of skin tests which uncover what substance(s) the child is allergic to. Some doctors consider such tests unnecessary, particularly in some regions of the United States, where allergens are extremely varied and contact is unavoidable in everyday life. Therapy for severe nasal congestion caused by allergic reactions may include the use of mucolytic syrups, which thin the mucous secretions and make them easier to expel, and/or special prescription inhalants that differ from the usual decongestant aerosols.

Other causes of nasal congestion include BACTERIAL INFECTION of the nasal-passage linings, often signaled by a discharge that is green or yellow; SINUSITIS, usually accompanied by headache or facial pain; and enlarged adenoids, which also causes snoring and mouth-breathing. Some infants will have nasal congestion when they are teething, and sometimes congestion occurs because a foreign body is lodged in the nasal passageway.

Nausea

An unpleasant, queasy sensation in the pit of the stomach. It can be caused by fright, anxiety, seeing or experiencing something upsetting, or as part of MOTION SICKNESS. Many youngsters will experience some degree of nausea at some point during most common childhood diseases. It can sometimes be relieved by having the child sip a mildly flavored carbonated drink, such as ginger ale, or letting him or her suck on crushed ice.

Although nausea usually precedes vomiting, it often occurs quite on its own.

Nearsightedness

A visual disorder called myopia, which occurs when the eyeball is too long from front to back. When light enters the eye, it is focused at a point in front of the retina. This causes a blurred image because the light rays disperse again before they actually reach the retina. Objects nearby can be seen far more clearly, which accounts for the name nearsightedness.

Unlike farsightedness, nearsightedness is rarely present at birth. It usually becomes evident in school-age children, who are seen holding books or other objects close to their eyes in order to achieve proper focusing.

The prevalence of myopia increases during childhood, peaking somewhere between the ages of eight and fourteen. So it is especially important for school-age children to have at least annual eye checks. If a school's screening program reveals any problem, the child should immediately be taken to an eye specialist so that appropriate corrective lenses can be prescribed.

Compare FARSIGHTEDNESS.

Neck stiffness

Many parents associate neck stiffness with dreaded diseases such as MENINGITIS or ENCEPHALITIS. But these diseases cause many other symptoms, such as high fever, severe headache, delirium, and the like, which alert parents to the child's need for immediate medical attention. Similarly, a disease such as JUVENILE RHEUMATOID ARTHRITIS is also accompanied by many other symptoms, including joint pain.

Most cases of neck-muscle discomfort reflect strains that occur as children play and fall, and simple rest and the application of warm compresses are all that should be needed. If the child suffers a severe accident and other symptoms are present, an emergency medical team should be called to move the child to a treatment facility.

Occasionally a spasm of the neck muscles many cause stiffness along one side of the neck without any known trauma. The head will be held tilted to the affected side, and the child will experience considerable discomfort if any attempt is made to straighten the neck. While the condition is most often caused by a strain, it can occur when a neck gland is infected. So a visit to the doctor is advised, especially if the child complains of sore throat or has a fever. If an infection is present, antibiotics will be prescribed. Otherwise, warm compresses, rest, and the use of children's dosage of aspirin or other pain-relievers will promote healing.

Nephritis

See KIDNEY INFECTIONS AND DISEASES.

Nephrosis

See KIDNEY INFECTIONS AND DISEASES.

Nervousness

A general term for an uneasy and/or agitated emotional state that can be behaviorally indicated by fidgeting, physiologically expressed by signs such as a fast pulse rate, and caused by factors ranging from a THYROID DISORDER such as an overactive thyroid gland to the presence of an ATTENTION DEFICIT DISORDER.

However, more often than not, nervousness is simply a transient sense of uneasiness such as adults, too, feel from time to time. Only when the frequency and degree seem grossly out of proportion to what is occurring around the child need parents be concerned. If supportive and reassuring discussion fails to reveal a cause and suggest a solution, it may be best to consult with a mental-health professional once the child's doctor rules out any physical cause.

Nightmares and night terrors

Sleep allows children to experience their own unconscious mind in a direct and uncensored way. Day-to-day happenings may be lived out in ways that cannot be perceived consciously or intellectually, and this relates very much to the child's level of cognitive and social development.

Children may not be able even to recognize, let alone discuss, fearful stresses such as new situations, school changes, dimly perceived family problems (even, for example, financial strain), or difficulties with some special age-peer friends.

Occasional nightmares and night terrors are rather common in children roughly between the ages of four and eight, probably for reasons mentioned in the previous paragraph. An episode of nightmare is rather fleeting, and sometimes children can tell his or her parents about the dream. In the case of night terrors, children may not quite awaken completely for a period of time, yet they cry out, look quite terrified, and may thrash about. They remain in what psychiatrists have termed a twilight state showing the appearance of experiencing great terror, still "seeing" frightening things, and not responding to the parents.

Holding and reassuring the child will, in time, usually provide sufficient comfort. If the child seems fearful of the dark, keeping a nightlight on may offer further solace. Children should remain in their own beds; they should *not* be allowed to sleep with their parents, which would reinforce the notion that something is unsafe and would also contribute to an unfortunate behavior pattern that may become difficult to change. Parents should *never* chase imaginary bears out of a closet or close shutters so ghosts can't come in the window. This only confuses children further, increasing the difficulty in differentiating reality from fantasy and making them wonder if, indeed, terrifying night creatures actually do exist.

Older children, particularly adolescents, can be expected to have nightmares that exaggerate their daytime worries of losing the next football game, missing a prom, failing an examination, losing the affection of a sibling or parent. Because of their greater cognitive and social development, adolescents usually have little trouble recognizing nightmares for what they are:

nightmares. They may even take some emotional comfort and some intellectual stimulation in discussing these dreams and analyzing what they represent.

Nipple, bleeding from

See BREASTS.

Nosebleed

Medically known as epistaxis, a nosebleed is one of the fairly common bleeding problems of childhood, although it is rare in infancy. Usually children's nosebleeds are caused by a rupturing of very small blood vessels in the nasal passageways. Common causes are injury, constant picking, nasal polyps (small growths), hay fever, and any number of infections. Nosebleeds tend to decrease in frequency as the child grows up.

Parents can take several measures to control the bleeding, including applying cold compresses to the bridge of the nose or using the thumb and forefinger to apply firm pressure to both sides of the affected nostril for five to ten minutes. During this time the child will be more comfortable sitting upright with the head slightly forward, to prevent blood from trickling down the throat.

If the bleeding cannot be controlled, take the child to a doctor or an emergency facility. Treatment may include packing with special cotton pads; the use of a drug that constricts blood vessels; and, in extreme cases, cauterization, a technique in which the doctor applies a substance or an electric current that blocks the source of the bleeding.

Adequate humidification of the child's room may help prevent future attacks, and children given to recurrent bouts of nosebleed should be discouraged from picking or rubbing their noses.

Most childhood nosebleeds are harmless. However, there is the possibility that they may indicate a more serious disorder such as high blood pressure, heart or blood-vascular disease, leukemia, or difficulties with the blood-clotting mechanism. So if the bleeding is severe and very frequent, a medical evaluation should be sought.

Nose, foreign body in

Young children sometimes insert foreign bodies into their noses and ears, probably as part of their curious exploration of body openings. Beads, dried peas and beans, and small stones are commonly used objects. Sometimes small wads of toilet or facial tissue are stuffed into nasal passageways.

The objects are generally impacted in the front section of the nose, so that they can easily be seen when a physician examines the child with an instrument called a nasal speculum. Removal, however, is a different story. A small, frightened child may rebel and create such a disturbance that anesthesia may have to be used. The physician needs to calm the child so that the object is not accidentally moved toward the back, where it may be carried down to a bronchus (one of the lung's major air passages).

Quite clearly, removal is not a procedure a parent should attempt. Also, while children need to be warned gently never to repeat this game, such a warning may not be necessary once they have endured retrieval procedures.

O

Obscene language

Four-letter words make their way into childhood vocabularies as a result of exposure to such language either at home or in peer groups. The two- or three-year-old who uses bad language usually hears it at home. Parental or older-sibling models who express anger with loud voices and cursing are indirectly telling the young child that it is acceptable to do this. Sometimes parents are so upset when their youngsters use obscene language that they curse back at the child, compounding the problem and reinforcing a vicious cycle.

On the other hand, young children will often come home from preschool, playgrounds, or schools and try out some four-letter word that they have heard but often do not even comprehend. This should generally be ignored, *certainly* not fussed about or unduly punished, such as by washing out a child's mouth. Parents may carefully but casually remark something to the effect that "In our family and among our friends, we prefer to use the word ———. Most people don't like vulgar words, and they often think poorly of people who use them."

Older children and adolescents may go through periods of swearing because it seems grown-up to them. They may also be trying to let you know that they are troubled by matters they are afraid to discuss, so using attention-getting bad language seems easier. Parents may be able to help by gently suggesting that they believe the young person has something on his or her mind and that perhaps discussing it—with the parents, or with a trusted outsider such as the family physician or another professional—would open new ways of coping with whatever is stressful.

When obscene language is associated with tics (involuntary blinking and muscular twitching) and violent jerking motions, one may suspect the presence of TOURETTE'S SYNDROME.

Obesity

See WEIGHT GAIN.

Otitis

See EAR INFECTION.

Outer ear infections

See EAR INFECTION.

P

Paleness

A loss of the normal brightness and tone of skin coloring, also called pallor. The child may look drawn, with circles under the eyes.

If the child is active and happy, parents need not worry. Sometimes fatigue causes changes in the appearance of a child's skin. During winter months when summer tans have faded and children spend most of their time inside home or school, a pasty color is common to many children's skin.

On the other hand, pallor may indicate any number of medical disorders: acute INFECTIONS, one of the many kinds of ANEMIA, excessive blood loss, lead poisoning, and LEUKEMIA, to name some of them. However, such conditions are also signaled by many other signs and symptoms. So in the absence of other problems, paleness in children should not cause parents undue concern.

Palpitation

Any throbbing, fluttering, or pulsating heart action the child is consciously aware of. The sensation is often associated with an unusually rapid HEART RATE. It generally lasts only a short time (usually a few seconds) and is ordinarily no cause for alarm. Sometimes palpitations can be a side effect of either a prescription or nonprescription drug.

If the condition persists, happens quite frequently, or worries the child, parents should arrange for a medical examination. In almost all cases palpitations will be tagged "functional," that is, having no organic or disease-related basis.

Panic attack

In a general way, anxiety may be differentiated from fear. The latter is usually aroused by some readily observable object, event, or set of circumstances that the child can understandably or justifiably perceive as frightening. Anxiety may occur in response to seemingly trivial things: a noise on the radio, a buzzing fly, a blinking light; or as a result of some inner experience of a physiological or psychological nature.

Because the autonomic nervous system—the one that controls involuntary processes like breathing—discharges or fires impulses so rapidly, the child may perspire, look pale, shake, and show rapid breathing and a fast heart rate.

Children stricken by this panic may feel dizzy or faint or numb, fear dying, or experience choking or smothering sensations. Occasionally they may fear that they are going crazy.

Calm reassurance may be of some help, but repeated episodes should warn the parent that a medical evaluation is needed. It has recently been found that these panic attacks may be associated with metabolic disease.

See also: FEARS.

Parental loss

See DEATH OF PARENT OR SIBLING.

Parental separation

With the increased frequency of divorce in the United States, many children must face the anxiety of losing their usual contact with one or the other of their parents. Custody battles, disagreements about visitation, and financial stresses make the child even more uncomfortable, and often the parents are so occupied with their own adult difficulties that they may be unaware of what the child is going through.

Often young children feel guilty because of the mistaken but almost unshakable belief that somehow they are to blame. They may fear abandonment by *both* parents and often try almost anything to bring the parents together again. Older children may have a somewhat better grasp of the situation, but they may develop a fear and avoidance of close relationships because they believe that other people, too, may leave them.

It may be helpful to discuss the whole matter with the children, on whatever level they indicate they are able to deal with it. Recriminations against the other parent should be avoided, and both parents should strongly reinforce the message that they love the children and that the split-up is *not* their fault. Both parents should also be sure they have someone else with whom they can discuss their own misgivings and anxieties, so that children are spared additional confusion. If a separation is inevitable, the process should not be dragged out, as the child needs to establish a sense of security within the new living arrangements as soon as possible.

If visitation rights are arranged, the schedule should be adhered to regularly. Consistency of contact and reassurance of continued parental love is much more important than frequency of visits. Failed visits reinforce whatever negative feelings the child may have.

When behavorial problems occur, they should be approached not from the standpoint of the behavior itself but with a view to the anxiety that most likely underlies the behavior.

Pediculosis

See LICE.

Penis swelling

If the foreskin is too tight and retracted back over the head of the penis, a compression may occur that causes considerable swelling and pain. Soaking the penis in warm saltwater may help reduce the swelling so that the foreskin can be gradually drawn forward.

Swelling may result from a bruise or bump against a hard object, such as might occur in a bicycle accident. Younger boys sometimes sustain a so-called ammonia burn from wet diapers or underclothing which may cause swelling. Healing and the prevention of further episodes are achieved by applying a protective cream or ointment as recommended by the local pharmacist or the family doctor.

Severe swelling of the penis demands prompt medical evaluation and treatment.

Peritonitis

Inflammation of the peritoneum—the thin, smooth, almost transparent, moist membrane that lines the walls of the abdominal cavity and parts of internal organs. The peritoneum provides a smooth surface upon which organs can glide as they undergo natural movement and slight changes of shape.

Before the advent of antibiotics, peritonitis was severely life-threatening. Even now it remains an extremely serious condition that requires immediate medical attention.

In children, the most common cause is a ruptured appendix. However, any condition that allows a spread of bacterial infection in the abdominal cavity can cause peritonitis. For example, a penetrating wound or a perforated large intestine may release bacteria-containing waste matter that can infect the entire peritoneal area. The infection can also be caused by the abnormal release of irritating body substances, such as bile, urine, blood, or digestive juices, into the abdominal cavity. Because female internal reproductive organs are so closely associated with the peritoneum, infections there can also spread.

The child with peritonitis may experience nausea and vomiting, fever, chills, abdominal bloating, and diffuse abdominal pain so severe that the slightest movement may make the pain worse. Muscular contractions that normally move intestinal contents may stop, so the child suffers constipation. A painful rigidity of abdominal muscles occurs because of the irritation inside the abdomen.

Once the parent has the slightest suspicion of peritonitis, absolutely no food and no laxatives should be given. The child's doctor or a medical emergency facility should be consulted immediately.

The child should be hospitalized so that antibiotics can be injected and nutrient fluids can be fed intravenously until healing occurs. If rupture or perforation of the intestinal tract or another body organ occurs, surgery is necessary to repair the affected organ.

Perspiration

See SWEATING.

Pertussis

Commonly called whooping cough, pertussis is a serious childhood disease, especially in babies under one year of age. The illness is a BACTERIAL INFECTION spread in the air from the breath or cough of an infected person; it is highly contagious. Complications such as pneumonia, inflamed intestines, and even convulsions can occur.

The first signs of whooping cough begin about one or two weeks after exposure to the germs. For several days or a week it seems to be just a bad chest cold with coughing. During the second week the coughing increases, coming in series of spasms between cough-free intervals. Children may cough several times very rapidly, "whooping" in an effort to catch their breath. The high-pitched, rasping sound is caused by air being sucked in over the vocal cords, which are covered with mucus. Spitting out some of the mucus relieves the attack for a time. Young infants are generally unable to clear this mucus. In fact, they may not show typical symptoms, such as whooping, but they are apt to suffer sudden bouts of extreme difficulty in breathing, whereupon they turn a bluish color.

Coughing and whooping may last for six weeks or more, but generally the intensity and frequency will taper after about the fourth week.

The child's doctor should be consulted promptly during the early stages of the illness. At times suctioning of mucus and oxygen therapy are required. In severe cases antibiotics may be prescribed, although they do not necessarily shorten the time a child has the disease. For the most part, tender loving care is the best treatment. The child's activity may be limited while symptoms are severe; later he or she can be up and about, although isolated from other children to whom the disease might spread. Feedings should be limited to frequent small helpings rather than large meals, and plenty of liquids should be offered, since they may help somewhat to thin the mucous secretions. In young children, solid foods should be restricted until the violent coughing begins to subside.

Children can be, and should be, protected from whooping cough by the DPT vaccination, one of the routine immunizations of childhood.

Pharyngitis

See SORE THROAT.

Phenylketonuria

Children with this inherited (genetically determined) disorder, often referred to by the initials PKU, are deficient in an enzyme that helps the body process an essential amino acid called phenylalanine. Amino acids are the building blocks of protein, without which normal growth and development are impossible.

Fortunately, screening for PKU in newborn babies is now an extremely widespread practice in developed countries; most states within the United States require it by law. Two popular PKU screening tests are the Guthrie bacterial inhibition test and the chromatography technique. Both start with a tiny sample of the infant's blood, usually obtained by pricking the heel. If the laboratory analysis shows an elevated amount of phenylalanine, more sophisticated diagnostic tests are done to confirm the diagnosis.

The child with phenylketonuria is placed on a special diet that provides little phenylalanine. Part of the diet is a milk substitute, such as LoFenalac. Fruits, vegetables, and other foods low in phenylalanine are also recommended. Many authorities now contend that this special diet can be altered or even discontinued altogether about the time the child is ready for school, convenient timing since as children become older, it is more difficult for parents to restrict their diets successfully.

When phenylketonuria is not detected and treated early, children are brain damaged by the excess chemical they cannot process. Symptoms of undetected PKU include mental retardation, seizures, and eczema (a generalized rash). Affected children usually have fair hair and skins, because phenylalanine inhibits the production of pigment; poor eating habits, with failure to thrive; and urine that has a peculiar odor.

PKU is a comparatively rare condition, occurring in about 1 in 10,000 births, but because it is a genetic defect, parents of a PKU infant may wish to seek genetic counseling about future plans for more children. PKU is carried by a recessive, not a dominant, gene. If two people both carrying the recessive gene choose to have a family, statistically, one-fourth of their children will have PKU; one-fourth will be entirely free of both the disease and the genetic trait; but one-half will themselves be carriers of the recessive trait for PKU, which means they could pass the disease or the trait to the following generation.

Phobia

See FEARS.

Physical disability

This entry is included, without definition, for a single but extremely important reason: children handle their physical disability precisely the way their parents handle it. If children are considered handicapped, they will consider themselves handicapped and increasingly refuse to try to do things that, with a little patience, they can learn to do.

If physically disabled children are reassured of their worth and receive consistently loving encouragement, they may find new ways to work around their limitations. Emotional support is also valuable in compensating for teasing by other children; it may even stop or prevent such teasing if the disabled child's conduct is self-assured.

Pigeon chest

A deformity, much less common than sunken chest, in which an overgrowth of breastbone-to-ribs cartilage causes an outward displacement of the chest.

In some infants the condition may be associated with congenital heart disease. Up to about age six, it may be associated with asthma. However, as a general rule, there is no interference with heart or lung functions, and there seems to be no definite cause for pigeon chest. Some cases appear in adolescence, when, with seeming suddenness, the chest wall may jut out some six inches or so.

If the deformity is severe, it will have very definite psychological implications. Cosmetic surgery can permanently restore normal chest contour, so if the child is of an age that a qualified surgeon agrees is appropriate, parents should give careful consideration to enhancing their child's chances for a life no longer marred by physical disability.

Compare SUNKEN CHEST.

Pimple

Any small, round swelling, usually red because it is inflamed, and which often exudes pus. A pimple may occur alone or in groups.

See also: ACNE.
Compare BOILS, CARBUNCLE.

Pink eye

See CONJUNCTIVITIS.

Pinworms

Also known as threadworms, pinworms are the most common worm infestation that children experience. In fact, especially in warm climates, pinworm infestation is an extremely common childhood ailment, and parents need not and should not feel it suggests household or personal lack of cleanliness.

At one time or another at least 20 percent of all children are infested with pinworms, which are harbored in the cecum, an intestinal pouch from which the appendix arises. The female worm travels down to the large intestine and rectum to lay her tiny eggs on the region around the anus. The eggs are passed to other individuals from hand contact with a contaminated object. Since children frequently put their hands in their mouths, spread is often easy after they have played with a toy or object that has eggs on it. The swallowed eggs go back down into the intestine, where they are hatched, and then the whole cycle is repeated.

Some children have no symptoms and signs, although occasionally abdominal pain, possibly mistaken for appendicitis, may occur. Many children recover spontaneously, provided reinfestation does not occur.

If children do have symptoms, they most likely complain of anal itching. This can become quite intense, and the whole area may become painful and reddened if the child scratches. Sleep, too, may be restless and uncomfortable, especially shortly after the child goes to bed.

Parents can use two methods to discover worms or eggs. After the child has been in bed asleep for a couple of hours, use a flashlight to examine the anal area. Pinworms are threadlike little creatures, quite small but visible to the naked eye. Another method involves using Scotch tape to pat the child's anal region. The strip of transparent tape, attached facedown to a glass slide, can then be taken to a lab or a doctor's office to see if eggs are present.

Pyrantel pamoate, piperazine citrate, mebendazole, and other anthelmintics (intestinal worm killers) are generally prescribed, and the doctor may choose to treat the entire family because the infection is so highly contagious. While some doctors suggest extra hygienic precautions, many authorities believe that meticulous standards of cleanliness, such as repeated hand-washing, have little effect on the control or prevention of pinworm infestation.

PKU

See PHENYLKETONURIA.

Pleurisy

Inflammation of the pleura (the membrane that covers the outside of the lungs and the inner side of the ribs).

Pleurisy is not particularly common these days, probably because it generally appears as a complication of some other condition such as rib injury or PNEUMONIA, which nowadays is usually effectively treated before pleurisy sets in.

The disorder called dry pleurisy begins suddenly with

very severe pain in the side, which becomes even worse when the child takes deep breaths, coughs, or moves. The pain is caused because the walls of the pleural membrane move against each other. A slight fever may be present. If the inflammation is mild, the pain will disappear in two or three days and the child will recover rapidly.

If considerable fluid builds up—a condition called pleurisy with effusion—there will be less pain because the walls of the pleural membrane separate, but shortness of breath may occur, and if the situation is left unattended, the excess fluid may cause collapse of a lung. The fluid may also begin to exude pus in a condition called purulent pleurisy, which can cause the child to cough up pus-tinged mucus.

When parents suspect pleurisy they should check with the child's doctor. In extreme cases it may be necessary to drain accumulated fluid.

Pneumonia

An inflammation of the lungs, typically accompanied by a collection of fluid in the alveoli (air sacs) or in the supporting tissues of the affected lung. Pneumonia can range from a small patch in one lung to extensive involvement of both lungs, called double pneumonia. Very mild and limited cases often go undetected and the child recovers completely.

Doctors classify pneumonia two ways: by the nature of the infection, usually viral or bacterial, and by the extent of the infection. Lobar pneumonia simply means that a major division of a lung, called a lobe, is involved. Bronchopneumonia has spread from a bronchus (one of the lung's major air passages), and an X ray will show a series of small solid patches of affected lung tissue rather than one large, dense area, as in lobar pneumonia. Influenza, acute bronchitis, pertussis, and measles are among the common predecessors.

Although less common than viruses or bacteria, causes can include fungi; the accidental inhalating of food particles, vomitus, or pus from an upper respiratory infection; or inhalating irritating gases or chemicals. Newborn babies occasionally contract pneumonia from aspirating meconium (a substance created in the baby's intestinal tract while the infant is in the uterus).

Babies born in a modern hospital have the advantage of immediate medical attention for this problem (as well as others), and the condition usually clears up without complications.

Pneumonia used to be extremely dangerous in young children. Currently, with prompt diagnosis and treatment, the child recovers often in less than a week, although general fatigue may keep him or her from normal activity levels for weeks to come.

Children with pneumonia can show quite different sets of signs and symptoms. Generally, however, they have had upper-respiratory symptoms such as a runny or stuffy nose for several days; fever and/or chills; a cough; and, occasionally, some chest pain.

Difficulty in breathing leads the child to take fast, shallow breaths; the nostrils might flare outward; the breathing may be accompanied by unusual noises; and, in severe cases, the skin takes on a bluish cast.

Once the diagnosis is made and appropriate antibiotics, and possibly an expectorant syrup, are prescribed, most children with pneumonia can be cared for at home. The child should try to rest until forty-eight hours after the shortness of breath, pain, and fever have gone. A full glass of nutritious liquid can be given every hour, which also acts to thin secretions and makes them easier to cough up. A cool steam vaporizer may be helpful.

If, of course, the child suffers from another disease or other diseases from which pneumonia can be a common complication, the child's doctor will recommend more stringent measures, which may include hospitalizing the child to monitor the condition more carefully.

Pneumothorax

A condition in which air escapes from the lungs and out into the immediately surrounding cavity, generally referred to as a collapsed lung. It can be caused by rupture of the lung or by some penetrating injury to the chest wall. In some newborn babies, especially premature infants on ventilators, weakness of the mid-chest may allow for enough tension to build so that pneumothorax develops. However, the hospital staff will be alert to diagnosis and appropriate treatment; complete recovery is the general rule.

Pneumothorax is certainly not a common disorder among children. However, because immediate medical attention is obviously required, parents should be alert to any sudden and unexplained development of breathlessness and pain or the complaint of a tight feeling in the chest, which worsens when the child breathes deeply. Severe shoulder pain may be experienced on the affected side. In one type of pneumothorax, in which the hole has sealed, symptoms may slowly disappear over a period of a few days.

Poisoning

Youngsters who have accidentally poisoned themselves can often be saved by prompt first aid. Adolescents who have taken poison in a suicide gesture or attempt, or who have overdosed on illicit or even legal drugs, may be expected to be uncooperative. Parents should not hesitate to call for police help in addition to contacting an emergency treatment facility.

In most instances of childhood poisoning, *prevention* is the key. Parents should take care to child-proof their home by keeping dangerous cleaning fluids or powders, plumbing solutions, and other such materials in safe places where curious youngsters cannot find them. Parents should also remember that many substances not generally thought of as being poisonous can readily poison a youngster who consumes too much. These substances include ordinary aspirin and other nonprescription painkillers.

First step: Purchase a bottle of syrup of ipecac at the local pharmacy. Activated charcoal liquid is also a useful antidote to many poisons. Some manufacturers have devised antipoison kits that contain measured doses of antidotes, along with specific instructions. Consider purchasing one of these kits and keep this material readily available.

Second step: Fill in the important phone numbers listed in the front of this book and also keep a list near a phone.

In the unfortunate instance that all child-proofing precautions are to no avail and an accidental poisoning occurs, call the Poison Control Center or the child's doctor for advice about what first-aid measures can be undertaken safely. Then immediately call for emergency medical assistance. When there is another adult or a responsible older child at home at the time, one does the phone-calling while the other performs first-aid measures.

If the child or adolescent is unconscious, there is nothing to do—that is, nothing you *should* do—until trained personnel arrive. On the other hand, if the child is conscious and vomiting must be induced or choking suppressed, here are some directions. If the child is not breathing but there is a pulse, perform some type of artificial respiration.

The following instructions are meant only as a brief guide to first aid. REMEMBER: TIME IS IMPORTANT; GETTING PROFESSIONAL HELP IS IMPORTANT.

Vomiting NOTE: if the child has taken lye or some other strong alkali, strong acids, cleaning fluid, or petroleum distillates such as kerosene, gasoline, coal oil, fuel oil, or paint thinner, do *not* attempt to induce vomiting unless the Poison Control Center, doctor, or other authority advises it. If vomiting is indicated, follow these instructions:

Do not use a salt-and-water solution.

Mix one tablespoon or ½ ounce syrup of ipecac with one cup water. Have the child drink this as quickly as possible, until vomiting occurs. Keep the child *facedown* with the head lower than the hips to prevent choking while vomiting. If no vomiting occurs within twenty minutes after the syrup of ipecac was given, repeat the same dose—but only once.

While the child is being transported to a medical facility, see that a sample of the vomitus is kept for examination. Also take along the poison container, with its label intact.

Artificial respiration For the mouth-to-mouth technique, clear the child's throat with your fingers. With the child lying down on his or her back, tilt the head straight back and breathe directly into the mouth until you see the chest rise. Then remove your mouth from the child's, allowing the lungs to empty. Keep repeating this at the rate of about twenty times each minute. If the victim is just an infant, blow shallow little puffs of air. Cardiopulmonary resuscitation (CPR) or external cardiac compression should be carried out simultaneously by another adult or older child who has been trained in the technique. The American Red Cross and other organizations frequently give training sessions for the general public, and at least one parent but preferably both should know how to perform this lifesaving procedure.

Parents are encouraged to read more about these vital

first-aid measures and to investigate their hometown's facilities for training in CARDIOPULMONARY RESUSCITATION.

Poison ivy, poison oak, and poison sumac

An acute inflammation of the skin with blistering, redness, and itching caused by contact with these plants. Direct contact is not always necessary; burning leaves that contain the oils of these plants can also spread the poison. Together these three plants create more cases of contact dermatitis than all other causes combined.

Prevention is the best treatment. When children or adults know they might come in contact with underbrush, they should be careful to wear long-sleeved tops, long pants, and high socks so there is less chance of exposure. Parents should know what these plants look like and teach their children which plants to avoid.

Poison ivy usually grows as a low shrub, but when support is available it climbs as a thick vine. The leaves are shiny, three to a stem, and have coarse serrated or toothlike edges. When cold weather approaches, there are clusters of white berries and the leaves change colors. Poison ivy thrives throughout the United States, except for those areas with very dry, hot climates.

Poison sumac, like the other shrubs in its family, may grow into a small tree. The stems are long, with shiny, small leaves arranged along either side and a single leaf at one end. Not nearly so widespread as poison ivy, poison sumac grows primarily in swampy areas.

Poison oak is not a tree, as the name might suggest. It resembles poison ivy, except that the leaves look like oak leaves. The climate along the west coast of the United States suits the plant well, and it is prevalent in that region.

Contact with the plant or the plant oils causes a reaction anywhere from six hours to six days later, usually in about two days. At first redness and itching develop. Because contact usually comes from brushing against leaves at a certain level, the irritation tends to develop in a linear pattern. Blisters soon appear, some of them very large, and the itching becomes intense.

Untreated, and if no secondary infection develops, the rash clears in two to three weeks. If there is a large amount of oil on the skin and the area is scratched, the inflammation can be spread. But, contrary to popular belief, fluid from ruptured blisters does not cause any problems.

Once contact has occurred the area should immediately be cleansed with soap (brown soap seems to work best) and water. The old remedy of allowing the brown soap to dry on the skin and then later washing again seems to offer some extra protection; it may absorb the oleoresin (the poisonous oil) before inflammation sets in. The child's clothes should be thoroughly washed or dry-cleaned.

Calamine lotion can reduce the itching of poison-ivylike rashes, but prolonged use may aggravate the problem by caking an accumulation on the skin. Hydrocortisone creams, now available without prescription, may speed healing. Antihistamines may also be useful, but they are apt to make the child drowsy.

If the child's doctor suggests the use of moist compresses, parents can prepare them at home by dissolving one packet of a special powder in a pint of cool tap water to make what is known as Burow's solution. In more severe cases that do not respond to home treatment, the child should be seen by a doctor. Short-term use of oral cortisone can provide dramatic relief.

Poliomyelitis

A viral disease, also known an infantile paralysis or polio, which may strike in the "minor-illness" category (with only slight symptoms and full recovery in about three days) or the "major-illness" category, which may affect the spinal cord and/or brain centers that control breathing and swallowing. In paralytic poliomyelitis, fewer than 25 percent of children affected suffer permanent damage to muscles such as varying forms of paralysis; some 25 percent have mild disabilities; and more than 50 percent recover with no paralysis. However, in children who contract bulbar poliomyelitis, in which breathing and swallowing are severely impaired, the use of artificial aids to respiration is generally required.

Early symptoms of polio include fever, headache, sore throat, and, sometimes, vomiting. Recovery may follow at this point. If it does not, the child may experience stiffness and pain in the neck and back, a warning that the disease may be progressing to its more serious, paralytic form.

The incubation period is from one to two weeks. If polio is even remotely suspected, the child should be put to bed immediately and kept there until medical help—sought on an emergency basis—is available. Activity during the early period of the disease may contribute to the development of paralysis.

Unlike parents of one and two generations ago, you need never worry about your children contracting poliomyelitis if you simply take advantage of the effective immunizations that are now common. Except in people over the age of sixteen, the original Salk vaccine, given by injection, has now been largely replaced with the Sabin vaccine, which is given by mouth in a liquid form or on a lump of sugar. Individual doctors differ somewhat in the scheduling of this immunization; some give the first dose when the baby is two months old, the second dose at four months, a booster dose at eighteen months, and another booster when the child nears school age. It can be given at the same time as DPT (diphtheria, pertussis, tetanus) injections, and parents are urged to consult the child's doctor about arranging for polio immunization.

There are no side effects to the vaccine, and afterward your child may eat and drink as usual and engage in all normal activities. It's been found that out of every 8.1 million immunizations, only one child contracts paralysis after they come into contact with the virus. That tiny risk seems far outweighed by the proven benefits of polio immunization for children. However, people who have not been immunized or who have an immune deficiency disease should avoid contact with an infant who has been given the oral vaccine; it is also possible to acquire the disease by viruses shed in the bowel movements.

Port wine stain

See HEMANGIOMA.

Postnasal drip

An increased secretion of mucus, part of which may drain down through the nose but most of which flows backward and is swallowed. For the most part, the child is not aware of the process, but if drainage is heavy, especially at night, he or she may experience a choking feeling and cough to try to clear the pooled secretions.

Under normal circumstances air is warmed as it passes through the nose. When children are heavily congested from postnasal drip, they breathe through their mouths and the cooler air irritates the throat. A vaporizer helps keep the drainage loose and flowing, and saltwater nose drops or sprays may help open the airway.

Postnasal drip is commonly caused by an ALLERGY, SINUSITIS, or UPPER RESPIRATORY INFECTION. If a BACTERIAL INFECTION is present, an antibiotic may be needed, so parents are advised to check with the child's doctor.

Posture

Unless some orthopedic problem such as SPINAL CURVATURE is present, parents and other adults should probably overlook children's slouching. Nagging does not improve the situation, and, generally speaking, when children grow older, become more aware of their appearance, and develop more self-confidence about their own bodies, they assume a better posture.

Children often try to make themselves more like their peers. For example, tall girls may tend to walk with their shoulders rounded and bent slightly forward so they don't tower over their friends. Short boys may swagger, with the shoulders thrown well back. Children tend to emulate their parents: if the father walks in an exaggerated masculine fashion or the mother takes mincing steps, children generally imitate these role models.

Pregnancy, teenage

A daughter's pregnancy in adolescence or a teenage son's responsibility for a girl's pregnancy may be the toughest issue a growing number of parents have to face.

Once pregnancy is a fact, and, for whatever reason, abortion is not a viable choice, the pregnant adolescent needs all the support, reassurance, and help her parents are able to give. Counselors experienced in this area are available to discuss keeping the child or arranging for adoption; whether the adolescent should remain at home during the pregnancy; whether a marriage is feasible and/or desirable; what arrangements can be made about school; and many other issues that *must* be decided on an individual basis.

There are many reasons teenagers become parents. Unfortunately, pregnancy in adolescence presents some potentially serious health problems to the young expectant mother and to her child, such as toxemia, a greater chance for premature delivery, and an increased incidence of congenital (present-at-birth) disorders. Therefore, it is important that the teenager receive adequate medical care if she desires to carry her pregnancy to term.

Prematurity

An infant born before full development within the uterus—which usually takes forty weeks or nine lunar months—is said to be premature. Before birth, special medical techniques such as ultrasound (a special kind of X-ray–type examination that measures sound waves) and amniocentesis (withdrawing and analyzing some amniotic fluid) may help to determine the infant's level of maturity. A fluid specimen withdrawn from the uterus may, for example, be tested to see if the baby's lungs are developed enough to allow survival without special respiratory-therapy measures.

Generally speaking, however, examination after birth is the best guide to assessing the premature infant's level of development.

All the important organs are basically formed by the sixth month of pregnancy, but they need more time to complete development. Premature babies have small stomachs, and they suck and swallow poorly. Their lungs need to be stronger, and they are especially prone to infections because their antibodies are not ready to defend them. The first twenty-four to forty-eight hours are the most crucial. The longer the pregnancy, the better the babies' chances for survival.

If the baby is more than five pounds, he or she may not need to be placed in an incubator. Smaller infants usually are. There the surroundings can be maintained much as they were in the mother's uterus, and because of the glass and plastic sides, doctors and nurses can keep a close watch. Premature infants may be given oxygen and fed by tube, and while in this special setting they can be weighed (a good key to whether the child is thriving), bathed, diapered, and otherwise taken care of.

As a rule of thumb, if the premature infant is born at two pounds, he or she is kept in the hospital for two months. Babies are generally discharged when they weigh about five and a half pounds.

Once home, a premature baby needs to be fed more often than a full-term baby; the nursery should be kept warmer than usual, and the doctor may suggest vitamins and an iron formula. Visits to the doctor may also be made more frequently than usual, possibly as often as every ten days for whatever period of time the doctor advises.

Parents of premature infants should not consider these children particularly fragile or in any way hampered. As the baby grows, he or she will catch up in terms of both size and general development. This is particularly true in the last quarter of the twentieth century, when an entire specialty—neonatology, the purview of neonatologists—has introduced highly specialized techniques and very sophisticated equipment into the prebirth, newborn, and early-infancy care of premature babies.

Prickly heat

See HEAT RASH.

Pruritus

See ITCHING.

Pulse rate

The number of pulsations felt over an artery (usually taken at the inside of the wrist or along the side of the neck). The pulse rate corresponds to the rate at which the child's heart beats.

See also: HEART RATE.

Pyloric stenosis

A thickening or overgrowth of the pylorus (the muscular ring) at the outlet of the stomach, which prevents normal flow of partially digested food into the intestines.

No one is sure what causes this disorder. It is more common in boys than in girls, and among firstborns, although the hereditary influence must not be strong, since later-born children in the family have only a slight tendency to have the condition more often than the average rate of occurrence than other children do.

Pyloric stenosis may be congenital (present-at-birth), but more often it develops over the first month or six weeks of life. Persistent vomiting is a common sign, and it may occur with sufficient force to propel the vomitus for some distance (called projectile vomiting). The baby's distended stomach can actually be observed to make forceful contractions in a futile effort to pass material beyond the blockage.

Occasionally doctors try special feedings and the use of an antispasmodic drug. However, surgical correction is very simple and is generally much more successful.

R

Rabies

A viral disease that attacks the nervous system; it is transmitted by bites of infected animals—dogs, cats, foxes, skunks, raccoons, and bats.

Any animal-bite wound should be cleaned first with soap and water and, if possible, let bleed a little. Then seek immediate medical attention. If possible, the animal should be captured and held for an examination by specialists. With prompt action, effective rabies vaccines can be administered.

Unfortunately, once symptoms appear, the disease is said to be invariably fatal. First symptoms are similar to those of influenza, followed by progressive irritability, anxiety, insomnia, and pain in the area of the wound. The rabies virus painfully constricts throat muscles if a victim attempts to drink water and swallow it. Heart and breathing muscles are paralyzed, and in the final stages a victim goes into violent convulsions, followed by coma and death.

See also: ANIMAL BITES.

Rectal bleeding

See BLOOD IN THE STOOLS.

Red streaks

See LYMPHANGITIS.

Regional enteritis

A disorder that mainly affects the small intestine and causes the lining to become inflamed, thickened, and less elastic.

It is not a particularly common disease, and it is extremely rare in children under the age of six. Despite the suggestion of a genetic defect, no definitive evidence for a hereditary basis has yet been discovered. Most authorities believe that emotional stress plays a definite role in causing and/or compounding the problem.

Many signs and symptoms may go on as long as three years before signs of intestinal inflammation can be detected by the child's physician. There is also wide variance from one child to another—some children experience sharp abdominal cramps or pains with recurrent attacks; occasionally the pains may mimic symptoms of acute APPENDICITIS; some children will be nearly incapacitated by the illness, which becomes chronic and may last into adulthood.

Most often the pattern is one of anorexia (diminished appetite), weight loss, nausea, abdominal pain, unexplained fever, diarrhea, and, at times, a hard mass that can be felt in the abdomen. At times the intestinal inflammation may be slight, but the thickness expands to form an intestinal obstruction that must be removed surgically. Another complication can occur if the affected area abscesses, walling off part of a perforated section of bowel and creating a fistula (an abnormal passageway to other bowel sections or out to the surface of the body).

To diagnose the condition the child's doctor has the youngster swallow a harmless white liquid containing barium. This material is opaque to X rays so that its progress through the intestinal tract is easy for the examining doctors to follow. A biopsy of the small intestine is sometimes done to confirm the diagnosis. Blood tests are also helpful in diagnosing and monitoring the condition.

If examinations confirm the diagnosis of regional enteritis various medications may be prescribed, such as antidiarrheals to decrease cramping and diarrhea; hydrocortisone to control inflammation; iron and vitamins to combat anemia or a nutritional deficiency; and antibiotics if infection is contributing to the problem. If medical management fails to correct the disorder, the child's doctor may recommend surgery to remove the diseased sections of intestine. While this is not a minor operation, it is quite safe in the hands of competent surgeons, and parents need not worry that it will impair their child's normal functioning and/or contribute to the development of other diseases later in life.

Regressive behavior

Behavior in which a child goes back to activities characteristic of a younger age, for example, a five-year-old starting to suck his thumb or wet his pants; a four-year-old reverting to the baby talk she outgrew two years earlier.

Usually such behavior is a coping mechanism, a means of dealing with stress experienced at the arrival of a new baby, the family's sudden need to move to a new location, or some other factor that observant parents can usually deduce. Generally speaking, parents are better off ignoring this temporary change in behavior. Scolding or mocking the child, for example, by making remarks such as "My, I thought you were four-and-a-half, not a baby," may act to reinforce the behavior as an attention-getting device.

If, however, the source of the child's stress cannot be determined and the regressive behavior continues longer than a week or two, parents may wish to seek professional advice, especially if the child also shows signs of EMOTIONAL WITHDRAWAL or DEPRESSION.

Restless behavior

Constant moving around or fidgeting, or a sleep disturbance usually induced by overexcitement or the experience of stress.

Boredom or the desire to be doing something else makes even the healthiest child restless, a phenomenon especially noticeable on rainy days or when children are almost but not quite recovered from an illness.

Only when restless behavior is associated with impulsivity, a short attention span, and extreme hyperactivity need parents suspect possible ATTENTION DEFICIT DISORDERS that demands professional assessment.

Reye's syndrome

A potentially fatal disorder that may affect children between the ages of five and fifteen who have recently been exposed to an acute viral infection such as influenza or chickenpox. It is characterized by severe disturbances of brain function, increased pressure on the brain, and fatty degeneration of the liver and other internal organs. In very mild cases, only about 20 percent of the cases prove fatal. In children whose illness progresses to convulsive seizures and respiratory arrest, the fatality rate may be over 80 percent. The overall average is slightly higher than 40 percent fatality.

Clearly, immediate medical attention and hospitalization are musts. Symptoms include persistent vomiting, high fever, headache, disorientation (lacking conception of time, place, and person), delirium, and fainting, possibly lapsing into coma.

Diagnosis is based on various laboratory findings that include increased ammonia levels in the blood; an abnormally low blood-clotting time; increased brain pressure as determined by examining cerebral spinal fluid; low blood sugar; and many measures of abnormal metabolism. Light-microscopy examination will show an accumulation of fatty deposits in internal organs.

Intravenous fluids are given in an attempt to correct any disturbance in body fluid/electrolyte (essential salts) balance. Intravenous administration of a diuretic (a medication that makes one urinate more frequently) may decrease pressure within the brain. Exchange transfusions (removal and replacement of the child's blood) may be done, and certain drugs, such as citrulline or nicotinic acid, may be used.

Rheumatic fever

A joint-inflammation disease that primarily affects children and adolescents. It strikes children from about age four to eighteen, but the majority of cases occur in children between eight and fifteen. Although the illness is often mild, rheumatic fever is a potentially serious condition. When it is left untreated it may scar the valves of the heart and lead to rheumatic heart disease, in which the valves are narrowed or otherwise kept from performing their normal work.

The exact cause remains unknown, although bacteria of the Group A hemolytic streptococci ("strep") type are involved, and the disorder generally appears within two to six weeks after a SORE THROAT caused by those germs. It is thought that the disease may represent an allergic reaction to bacterial toxins. The antibodies formed (as a result of the allergic reaction) in turn inflame normal body tissues including the heart and joints.

After the sore throat or other upper respiratory infection, symptoms include pain, stiffness, and swelling in one or more of the large joints: shoulder, elbow, wrist, hip, knee, or ankle. Smaller joints are rarely affected. The pain may last only a day or so in a particular joint before it moves on to another. This contrasts with arthritis, in which the pain is more constant in one joint. Other signs and symptoms include fever (which may not be very high), rapid pulse, sweating, and possible pallor (paleness), nosebleeds, and weight loss. Weakness, difficulty breathing, feeling very tired, and possible chest pain may occur with heart involvement. In some cases emotional upset and aimless muscle movements may appear. Sleeping may be difficult if the child is experiencing fairly severe joint pain.

Because many children suffer only mild symptoms, rheumatic fever may go undiagnosed. At best, diagnosis is based primarily on the presence of several symptoms and signs, as well as evidence of a recent strep infection. There is no single test that establishes the disease's presence; some laboratory findings mimic those of other diseases.

The child's doctor will usually suggest aspirinlike drugs to lower fever and reduce inflammation; he or she may also prescribe antibiotics to wipe out any remaining streptococcal infection and, if necessary, digitalis or other cardiac drugs to treat any heart symptoms. Sometimes hospitalization will be recommended during the acute phase, partly to permit more careful monitoring.

In the majority of cases, recovery is complete. In fact, in about half of the patients who are found to have some form of chronic rheumatic heart disease, there is no clear medical history of their having had rheumatic fever.

See also: ENDOCARDITIS.

Rh problems

An adverse reaction between a mother's blood and the blood of her unborn baby.

The Rh factor is a special factor in the blood. It gets its

name from the first two letters of *Rhesus monkey,* animals with which experimental work was done. If the mother is Rh-negative and the fetus inherits red blood cells of the Rh-positive type from its father, antibodies may be formed. Antibodies are types of body proteins intended to combat foreign substances; in this case, antibodies react against the baby's own red blood cells. These antibodies may cross back and forth across the placental barrier, so that future infants, too, can be affected by the antibodies in the mother's circulation.

Problems may start while the infant is still in the uterus; after birth, ANEMIA and JAUNDICE may occur, as well as seizures, extreme difficulty in breathing, hearing loss, and mental retardation. Very severely affected infants may die shortly after birth; some die while they are still in the uterus.

Fortunately, modern medical methods permit early detection of this incompatibility. Both the mother's and the father's blood can be tested so the doctor can be alert to the possibility of Rh problems. The mother can be tested and carefully monitored throughout pregnancy. By a process called amniocentesis, material can be withdrawn from inside the birth sac and various analyses can be made to determine how the developing baby is doing.

When an Rh incompatibility exists, the newborn baby is given various blood tests and probably an exchange transfusion of blood. Phototherapy (light therapy) with special fluorescent lights is another treatment used. If appropriate treatment is administered immediately in the newborn period, the baby develops his or her own blood type and no long-term ill effects will remain from the Rh incompatibility.

Rickettsial infection

Any infection caused by Rickettsia (extremely small parasitic microorganisms about midway in size between bacteria and viruses).

They usually attach themselves to insects and then may be passed on to human beings by insect bites. Such diseases include Rocky Mountain spotted fever, Q fever, and typhus.

Infected children usually show fever and skin rashes. A doctor's diagnostic laboratory tests include measurement of the rise of antibodies that specifically fight Rickettsial infections. Treatment is by use of a broad-spectrum antibiotic.

Ringing in the ears

See TINNITUS.

Ringworm

A fungus infection of the skin, hair, or nails. It has nothing to do with worms but is named after the ringlike lesions produced.

School-age children and adolescents are particularly prone to contract tinea corporis (ringworm of the body) from floors and shower stalls or benches contaminated with fungi. Pet cats may have facial ringworm lesions that are not noticeable but prove a source of infection to owners who nuzzle their pets.

Treatment may include scrubbing with skin cleansers such as Betadine; application of antifungal creams; keeping the skin dry; and carefully avoiding any exchange of contaminated clothing, towels, and linens, which should be boiled or chemically sterilized.

Tinea capitis (ringworm of the scalp) can be transmitted by the practice of exchanging hats and brushes; by barbers' or hairdressers' instruments; even by leaning against theater seats. Boys are somewhat more susceptible than girls.

The disorder is painless, but it causes some patchy hair loss and split hairs, inflammation, and scaling. On occasion treatment may require the use of oral griseofulvin-type antibiotics in addition to the measures previously described.

Rocking

A form of motor activity in which the infant or young child rocks to and fro, especially before going to sleep. The rhythmic movement seems to induce relaxation, although at times it may become quite forceful and include HEAD BANGING.

Many children who rock excessively seem to be more easily agitated by noise and movement around them than other children are. Cutting down on these stimuli may decrease the rocking. Older children engage in this behavior less often if they are allowed to do it by more socially appropriate means, as in a small rocking chair.

Roseola

A viral infection most commonly seen in infants under the age of one year.

The youngster may show a fever as high as 105°F without having many other symptoms. This is generally alarming to parents, but the illness is benign and usually goes away by itself within a week.

The baby may seem droopy when the fever is at its highest, but when it is around 102° or 103°F he or she may play and smile. Elevated temperatures usually break after four or five days, and, unlike other viral rashes, it is after the fever breaks that the reddish rash appears, only to fade in about a day.

The nasal congestion that usually accompanies roseola may lead to an ear infection; otherwise there is no need for concern except to alert the parents of other babies the infected infant may have come in contact with to the possibility that their child may have caught the infection.

Roundworm

See ASCARIASIS.

Rubella

An acute viral disease, also known as German measles, that is a much milder disease of childhood than true MEASLES. It is also much less contagious than "red" measles, although it, too, is spread by viruses from the nose and throat of an infected person. The incubation period is about two to three weeks.

First signs and symptoms are sore throat, low-grade fever, mild upper-respiratory symptoms, muscular aches and pains, some stiffness of the neck, and some swelling of glands in various parts of the body, particularly below and behind the ears.

The rash, consisting of small, flat, pink spots, may appear first on the face and neck and then spread to the trunk and the limbs.

Parents should call the doctor for a confirmation of the diagnosis, but rubella is essentially a home-treatable disease. Make sure the child gets plenty of rest, eats lightly, and is given cooling drinks. If itching becomes bothersome, the child can be bathed in cool water. Medicines are generally not needed and should not be given without checking with the child's doctor.

One attack of German measles usually provides protection for life. It is only in adults that the disorder may be more serious; this is especially so in the case of unimmunized pregnant women, because it can affect the unborn child.

Running away

Around the ages of six to eight, when children are tasting their first trips on their own (perhaps going to school by themselves) and flexing their imaginations about what they are capable of doing, "running away from home" is not at all unusual. Parents generally consider it unusual only when it is discovered. They often don't *know* that their children did it until then, and/or they forget about the time they themselves may have bundled together some provisions and gone all of three blocks until they and their friends decided the North Pole was simply too far.

On the other hand, if a child does this consistently over a period of time, then even these childish escapades merit some discussion. Explore the child's own reasons and feelings about wanting to run away. What might be missing in the home life parents are providing? What is it that the child is really seeking? Good parenting often requires some change in the parents' own behavior.

Runaway teenagers present quite another problem. About a million American adolescents leave home each year, many with the intention of never returning. This escape may reflect a parental lack of support, whether perceived or real; feelings of rejection; self-doubt about their own worth and lovableness.

Parents might want to call the adolescent's close friends for clues to a destination. If you're sure the child has fled, do not hesitate to report it to the police no matter how embarrassing this may be. Stay calm, for the search may take weeks. Most teenagers, however, do not go far, and the majority of runaways return within two weeks. If the runaway teenager phones, parents should not respond with anger and blame, which only reinforces the negative feelings that provoked the teenager's leaving. It is important that parents reassure the adolescent of their love, concern, and desire that he or she return home so the family can work this out together. When the reconciliation occurs, parents must be sure to make good on their promise to work things out together. Professional counseling is often helpful through providing an outside, more objective mediator.

See also: DEPRESSION, EMOTIONAL WITHDRAWAL.

Ruptures

See HERNIA.

S

Salmon patch

See HEMANGIOMA.

Scabies

A red skin rash, which develops bumps, blisters, and red tracks, marked by extremely intense itching.

Scabies is caused by small, insectlike organisms called mites, which burrow into the skin. A doctor makes the diagnosis by removing the parasite with a needle and then examining it under a microscope.

Contrary to popular opinion, this infection is not limited to individuals who live in crowded, unsanitary habitats. It is, however, highly contagious, and if the child is infested, the entire family should be examined and treated. Bed linens, towels, and clothing should be dry-cleaned or washed in very hot water, then ironed with a hot iron.

Scabies usually develops about four to six weeks after exposure. The rash may appear all over the body, but body folds, such as between the fingers and toes, under the arms, in the groin, or behind the knee, are particularly susceptible. Infants often show the rash on their face and neck. Scratching causes small scabs, hence the name *scabies,* and it can also cause skin scrapes that become infected by bacteria.

Treatment generally consists of cutting the child's nails short to discourage scratching, use of an antiseptic soap in hot tub soaks, application of various creams or lotions containing a chemical such as lindane, and, if there is bacterial infection, an antibiotic. The child should be kept home, away from school and/or playmates, for 24 hours after treatment has been instituted. Following that brief period, full social contact can be resumed.

Scalds

See BURNS AND SCALDS.

Scarlet fever

Any child with a sore throat caused by streptococcal infection and a fine, slightly raised, scarlet-colored rash that begins on the neck and behind the ears and then spreads rapidly over the entire body is said to have scarlet fever.

A throat culture is necessary to confirm the presence of a strep infection. Modern antibiotic therapy successfully treats this contagious bacterial infection.

The incubation period is from one to five days; the contagious phase usually starts a day or two before symptoms begin. Children are no longer contagious after they have been treated with an appropriate antibiotic for 24 hours.

The first signs are common to many other illnesses: sore throat, chills, fever, cough, and sometimes nausea and vomiting. The tongue may be covered with a white coating that gradually peels off to show a bright-red strawberry tongue. About a day later the rash usually breaks out, and about a week later small, round patches of dead skin flake off.

In addition to giving the child whatever medication the doctor prescribes, parents can offer cooling drinks and basically keep the youngster comfortable.

Scars

The natural repair of injured tissue. Scars appear anywhere on or in the body, but the tendency is to think in terms of skin wounds.

Depending on the extent of the injury, scar formation may take many months, and the tissue changes appearance. At first the injured area appears reddened and the scar line seems relatively wide. Gradually the area whitens as the tissue under the injury builds strength. Eventually the rough and uneven surface draws back, and the scar assumes its true size and color.

Children are especially prone to many accidents that leave scars, especially around the knees, legs, and, to a somewhat lesser extent, arms. Faces and heads and lips are not immune, although modern techniques of clamping or suturing may make such scars almost invisible.

Unless scars are genuinely disfiguring they probably should be ignored.

School failure

See UNDERACHIEVEMENT.

Scoliosis

See SPINAL CURVATURE.

Seizure disorders

A seizure is an episode of uncontrolled motor activity, usually involving jerking movements, especially of the extremities, and some alteration in consciousness (often, but not necessarily, the loss of it). All these seizure disorders, often called convulsive disorders, involve some disorganization or disruption in the normal flow of nervous impulses coming from the brain.

Epilepsy. If seizures occur before a child is two, the condition is usually connected to some birth injury, developmental defect, or metabolic disease. In epilepsy affecting children between two and fourteen, no definite cause can be found in more than two-thirds of cases. Heredity has long been thought to play a role, but its precise influence has not been fully determined.

Grand mal seizures, also called generalized seizures, are typically preceded by an *aura:* a personal kind of warning system that may be sensed as some vague sensation, images and thoughts, or gut feeling. The aura lasts only about a minute, after which the child usually makes a throat gurgle and then exhibits jerking, twitching convulsions of the whole body. Bladder and bowel control may be lost, drooling may occur, and the child may even turn blue. The seizure itself may last several minutes. Afterward the child is likely to fall into a deep sleep.

In petit mal seizures, the child may seem to stare and then twitch, blink, or nod during a five- to thirty-second lapse of consciousness. If undiagnosed, the condition may lead to other problems, because these children are not aware of the lapse of consciousness and, for example, teachers and other children may conclude that they are inattentive.

Diagnosis of epilepsy has been greatly aided by electroencephalogram (EEG) examinations, skull X rays, lumbar punctures (for examining cerebrospinal fluid), CAT scans, and laboratory analyses of serum glucose and calcium levels.

Prescription drugs such as phenytoin and phenobarbital can totally control grand mal seizures in about half the children affected and can greatly reduce them in an additional one-third. Other prescription drugs effectively combat both grand mal and petit mal seizures.

Parents and others should know how to prevent injury, for example, by inserting a firm (but not *too* hard) object between the child's teeth to prevent tongue damage. For example, a stick would do. Clothing around the neck should be loosened, and a pillow may be placed under the child's head.

Psychomotor seizures. This condition is characterized by automatic behavior, such as lip smacking, running around in circles, or uncontrollable crying or laughing for no perceptible reason. The defect is focused in the temporal lobe of the brain. Extremely careful diagnosis and medical treatment are necessary to control the disorder because, later on, it may lead to violent and potentially dangerous outbursts.

Minor motor convulsions. Infants and toddlers may exhibit seizure episodes in which the head suddenly drops to the chest, the legs come up toward the stomach, and the arms are drawn over the chest. Sometimes small areas of muscles twitch, and sometimes a toddler may seem to be performing some purposeful activity, like a fancy, twisting fall, before parents are aware it is a seizure. Afterward the child may be unconscious or drowsy.

Insofar as is possible, children with seizure disorders should be encouraged to lead a normal life. Overprotection may deepen the affected child's sense that he or she is inferior and handicapped. If retardation exists, special-education programs can be helpful. Generally speaking, intelligence is not affected, nor do the seizures permanently damage the brain.

Frequent medical checkups are a must so that medications can be adjusted and the child's progress can be followed.

Parents should understand that the general subject of seizure disorders covers many different kinds of conditions beyond those mentioned here and elsewhere in this book, such as FEVER CONVULSIONS. A more detailed discussion is beyond the scope of this book; besides, the field is so highly specialized that both the child and the parents are best served by consulting with appropriate medical specialists who can explain the particular seizure disorder and outline individualized methods of treatment and control.

Self-exploration, self-manipulation

See MASTURBATION.

Septicemia

Commonly known as blood poisoning, the condition occurs when the bloodstream is invaded by disease-causing bacteria and their toxic by-products.

This condition should be treated as a medical emergency. Parents should take the child to a doctor or an emergency facility at once, for children with untreated septicemia can die within hours.

The child's symptoms may include the abrupt appearance of high fever, chills, irritability, sometimes delirium, and later with extreme lethargy or even prostration. In severe cases vascular (blood-vessel) shock may ensue, so that blood pressure decreases; the child shows a fast but feeble pulse; the respiratory rate is slowed; paleness or a bluish coloring may occur; skin will be sweaty and clammy; and stupor, unconsciousness, or coma can occur. A purplish body rash may develop quickly, which indicates the leakage of blood through small vessels.

Sexual abuse, molestation

The child who has been sexually abused undergoes special trauma because sexuality is undefined, poorly understood, confusing, and often scary.

Parents may compound this problem and unwittingly contribute to the potential for hampered sexual maturing by too loudly expressing their anger, fear, distaste, and vindictiveness toward the guilty party. An air of calm and support should prevail, especially when reporting the crime and during the offender's prosecution. The parents and child may find themselves walking an emotional tightrope after the attack. To help the child avoid dwelling on the event, parents and others should not dwell upon it, most especially in the child's presence. However, the event should not be ignored. Allow the child to talk about the incident as and when he or she wishes. If marked emotional difficulties ensure, the child needs supportive counseling by professionals who specialize in working with victims of sexual abuse.

Suggestions for reporting incidents of child molestation are outlined under INCEST.

Sexual development, premature

Hormonal changes at puberty cause the development of what are termed secondary sexual characteristics: male or female distribution of body hair; breast enlargement in the female; enlargement of the testicles and penis, as well as voice changes, in the male.

On occasion, signs of secondary development may be noticed in very young children. A two- or three-year-old girl may show breast enlargement. A little boy may develop pubic and armpit hair without showing any growth in the size of testicles. Secondary sexual characteristics can be considered premature if they occur in a girl younger than eight and a half or a boy younger than ten—approximately three years earlier than the average ages at which such changes occur. The situation may arise because of premature production of hormones in the brain, the ovaries or testes, adrenal glands, and, in a few cases, the liver. More often, the usual cause is an unusual sensitivity of the end organ (breasts, skin, etc.) to normal levels of circulating hormones. The changes are essentially harmless, but the child certainly should be evaluated by a physician to make sure there is no underlying disease contributing to the early development. At times professional counseling may be needed if the child becomes unduly disturbed by these bodily changes. Parents should remember that roughly from the age of eight or ten well into adolescence, children want very much to be like their peers. Thus a boy in intermediate school may be more embarrassed by than proud of his bass voice.

Sexual preoccupation

A child's inordinate attention to sexual matters.

This preoccupation usually stems from anxiety about sex or even about entirely different matters. Some authorities believe it can be stimulated by viewing explicit sexual material, observing parents or other adults during intercourse, or witnessing nudity in the household.

Children are quite normally curious about sex and their own sexual feelings, but facing these issues before they are sufficiently mature may cause considerable confusion and emotional discomfort. Instead of running from the subject, some children become fascinated, further stimulated, and then quite preoccupied. They should not be teased or punished, but they should be encouraged to discuss their feelings and their fears on whatever level the *child* indicates is comfortable. If the problem cannot be solved at home, the parents and the child may benefit from some professional counseling.

Shin splints

Intense discomfort of the lower leg(s), usually after heavy exertion, although some individuals may develop pain after a short walk. It is uncommon in childhood but may be seen in 5 percent of adolescents, especially among athletes. The pain is thought to come from an inflammation of muscle attachments to bone. If the muscles are chronically misused, there may be tears of the muscle fibers, and it is this injury that results in the pain and tenderness.

Although many cures are offered, the only effective therapy is rest, avoiding running, or the activity that causes the pain until there are no symptoms. This rest period should be at least five to seven days. The next step is avoidance of the activity completely or a change in the child's approach to it. A gradual buildup may help, as may altering the speed, amount of exertion, or even the surface on which any running takes place. Improper footwear may strain lower-leg muscles, causing a greater tendency to develop shin splints.

Another defect, called anterior tibial compartment syndrome and less frequent than shin splints, develops because the compartment enclosing the lower-leg muscles is tighter than it should be. If activity causes sufficient swelling in the lower-leg muscles, there may be enough pressure built up to press on arteries that supply the lower leg and foot. Usually rest relieves the symptoms, but if tingling or weakness of the ankle or foot develop, an urgent medical evaluation is advised. If symptoms of leg pain last longer than ten to fourteen days, a fracture may be present, such as a stress fracture, and an X ray is needed for diagnosis.

Shock

A type of collapse caused by an extreme deficiency in blood circulation, depriving body tissues and organs of oxygen.

Shock may be caused by injuries and burns, various kinds of poisoning, acute infections, inflammations of internal organs, heat stroke, hemorrhage, ANAPHYLACTIC SHOCK (a life-threatening allergic reaction), and other factors that interfere with normal circulation.

A child in shock may show a low body temperature, cold and clammy skin, shallow breathing, a fast but weak pulse, thirst, vomiting and diarrhea, and a general picture of complete prostration.

Shock is a medical emergency. Treatment may consist of intravenously administered solutions, oxygen inhalation, and the use of drugs. The child in shock should immediately be wrapped in a blanket and taken to an emergency facility if a mobile unit cannot promptly be dispatched to the home.

Shingles

See HERPES ZOSTER.

Shoulder pain

Like all body joints, the shoulder may become painful if its surrounding ligaments are strained. Chronic misuse of the arm—from activities such as throwing a ball too hard and for too long a time, excessive baton-twirling practice, even too-vigorous bowing of a violin—is the commonest cause of shoulder pain in children.

Generally, rest and the soothing application of moist heat brings relief. However, if the pain is accompanied by redness and a fair degree of swelling, parents should check with the child's doctor. It is possible that an inflammatory disease such as JUVENILE RHEUMATOID ARTHRITIS may be present, or, in very rare cases, a bacterial infection of the joint itself. If the child is acutely short of breath, shoulder pain could be a symptom of PNEUMOTHORAX. If fever and cough accompany the shoulder pain, PNEUMONIA might be present in the lower part of the lung.

Sibling loss

See DEATH OF PARENT OR SIBLING.

Sibling rivalry

The child's feeling, whether real or only perceived, that another child in the family is more favored by the parents.

There is probably no way to stop all squabbling among children within a family. Indeed, unless such fighting gets out of hand, it may prove somewhat beneficial in teaching children to negotiate, compromise, and manage to get along with other people. Parents can, however, definitely help dissuade their children from believing they are less favored and/or from constantly battling for parental attention and love.

Everyone needs privacy. If separate rooms are not possible, areas within the house or bedroom(s) should be designated for each child. Each child should also be regularly given his or her time alone with each or both parents. This should be a time for relaxation, shared conversation, and a discussion of feelings when the child is free from interference by siblings.

Older siblings should be given greater privileges, but increased responsibilities should accompany the increased freedoms. Similarly aged children should be disciplined in the same way. If a parent is confused about who started a fight, either both children or neither child should be disciplined. Parents should strive to treat each child as an individual, so that any special needs can be defined and then met.

SIDS

See SUDDEN INFANT DEATH SYNDROME.

Sight

See BLURRED VISION, DIABETES MELLITUS, DOUBLE VISION, FARSIGHTEDNESS, NEARSIGHTEDNESS, STRABISMUS.

Sinusitis

Inflammation of the mucous-membrane lining of the sinuses (drainage channels), partly filled with air, in the facial part of the skull.

Infants and very young children have only two pairs of the total of four pairs that eventually develop. Therefore, their signs and symptoms may differ from the complaints of older children.

Pain occurs when the inflammation swells narrow openings into the nose, so that pressure builds up against the bony walls of the sinus. X rays will help identify a blocked sinus, which will appear dense because it is filled with fluid rather than air.

Babies and youngsters may show swelling of the skin surrounding the nose and eye. They may seem to have one cold after the other, or a cold that never goes away. Older children may complain of headaches, an aching behind the eyes, or tooth pain. Fatigue, a chill, changes in weather, or contact with allergy-stimulating substances may aggravate the condition. Nasal congestion and other symptoms, such as a cough, may resemble the effects of a bad cold; indeed, acute sinusitis frequently follows a cold or other upper-respiratory infection.

A doctor's treatment may include prescription nose drops, washing out of the affected sinuses, and, in severe cases, a small incision to allow for proper drainage. An antibiotic will be prescribed if a bacterial infection is present. Signs of such an infection include a cough that will not go away, fever, a runny nose, and a persistent postnasal drip. Pus may be present in the nasal discharge.

Parents can help provide relief by applying moist-heat compresses; using a vaporizer in the child's room; encouraging the child to drink plenty of liquids, which may help thin secretions; and, if the doctor advises, giving children's doses of aspirinlike painkillers. If the youngster can't blow his or her own nose, the doctor may instruct parents on how to use a nasal aspirator to suction each nostril gently after nose drops have been given.

Skin infection

Any inflammation of the skin caused by fungi or by a BACTERIAL INFECTION. Streptococci and staphylococci are usually involved, entering through small breaks in the skin. The most common of the bacterial infections that affect children's skin is IMPETIGO.

Skin rashes

A redness or eruption on the skin. Skin rashes are frequently associated with childhood illnesses such as chickenpox and measles, but they may also be associated with more serious diseases or with direct bacterial infection.

See also: ALLERGY, CHICKENPOX, CRADLE CAP, DIAPER RASH, ECZEMA, FIFTH DISEASE, HEAT RASH, HEMOPHILIA, IMPETIGO, MEASLES, ROSEOLA, RUBELLA, SCABIES, SKIN INFECTION.

Sleep problems

A disturbance of the normal sleep process involving inability to get to sleep, constant awakening, getting out of bed and wandering about, difficulty falling back to sleep. All the problems qualify as insomnia.

Most sleep problems in children can be prevented by consistent behavior on the part of the parents. Bedtimes should be established and followed. Certain bedtime rituals may help: tucking in, bedtime stories, a brief conversation about the day's events, or, for babies, some gentle patting.

See also: NIGHTMARES AND NIGHT TERRORS, SLEEPWALKING.

Sleepwalking

A sleep disturbance in which the child walks around even though he or she is not alert or fully awake. It is somewhat more common in boys than in girls, and the fact that it is frequently outgrown suggests more of a maturational than an emotional basis.

Parents may wish to take precautions around the house such as installing a gate at the tops of stairways in a multilevel home and being sure that windows and exterior doors are locked. The child's bedroom door should *never* be locked from the outside in case of fire or some other emergency. A screen door may be trimmed to fit the child's bedroom door, which will allow parents to look in and the child to look out or call out and be heard if need be.

Although sleepwalking is usually harmless and, incredibly, most children do not hurt themselves while in this state, the phenomenon can on occasion signal some psychiatric or medical difficulty. So if the problem persists over a long period of time or the child shows evidence of other problems, he or she should be checked by a qualified physician.

Smallpox

An acute, highly contagious, disfiguring, and potentially fatal disease caused by infection with a virus.

Fortunately, the disease has been conquered by the World Health Organization's worldwide vaccination campaign launched in 1967. Since 1982 the disease is considered essentially eradicated.

Because of this progress, the fact that there has been no case in the United States or Canada reported since 1949, and the view of many doctors that the complications from vaccination may now outweigh its benefits, children in the United States are no longer required to be vaccinated as a routine precaution.

However, if children have been exposed or are traveling to an area that is still at high risk, their doctors may recommend vaccination. After receiving the vaccination most children show some slight fever and perhaps swelling of the lymph glands, and they may complain of a headache. Aside from encouraging the child not to scratch the site, parents need do little except keep the child away from anyone who has open sores, as the vaccination site can easily become infected by other viruses or bacteria, and perhaps covering the spot with loose gauze to prevent its being rubbed by clothing. About two weeks after vaccination a crust forms over what started as a firm red spot and then develops a blister in which clear fluid turns into a thick, yellow fluid resembling pus—all of which indicates that the vaccination has "taken." The crust should not be removed. It will fall off by itself.

The doctor need not be consulted again unless the child develops a temperature higher than 103°F, a skin rash appears elsewhere, or the vaccination does not take.

Smoking

In current parlance smoking applies mostly to the use of marijuana. There is considerable controversy about results of its habitual use, but children and adolescents should be reminded that altered mental functioning and impaired physical reflexes provide the potential for extremely dangerous accidents, such as fatal automobile crashes.

See also: CIGARETTE SMOKING.

Snake bites

Only a few snakes common to North America secrete an amount of venom sufficient to cause potentially serious problems in a child who is bitten.

There are at least two schools of thought about snakes: one is to consider all of them possibly dangerous and seek immediate medical attention if bitten. The other recommends learning the characteristics of poisonous snakes that inhabit your locality and being prepared to render first aid in the event that aid is not readily accessible.

Many varieties of rattlesnakes, water moccasin, and copperhead snakes are known as pit vipers because they have a pit between the eyes and nostril and on each side of the head. Their heads are rather flattened, their pupils have an elliptical shape, and they have two well-developed fangs. Two very clear puncture wounds are left where the fangs enter the skin.

Coral snakes are cobras. They have a black nose; red, black, and yellow rings around the body; and their fangs are tubular, with teeth behind the fangs. They tend to hang on to the victim, chewing into the skin.

The bite of a coral snake tends to be somewhat less painful than bites by pit vipers, and there is less immediate swelling. Other than that, symptoms are similar: weakness, shortness of breath, impaired vision, rapid pulse rate, nausea, vomiting, and, in severe cases, possible shock, respiratory problems, convulsions, paralysis, and coma.

First-aid procedures. The best treatment is immediate medical attention so that an appropriate antivenom substance can be administered. Personnel in most hospital emergency rooms no longer incise (cut) such wounds, and the effectiveness of tourniquets is in question. However, when a delay in getting modern medical treatment is unavoidable, these first-aid steps may prove valuable:

1. Immobilize the bitten area in a position lower than the heart and apply a constricting band just tight enough so that you can slip a finger under it between 2 and 4 inches above the bite, that is, between the bite and the heart.
2. Use a flame to sterilize a sharp knife, then make a short cut (no longer than ½ inch) in an up-and-down direction (*not* crossways) where the venom seems to be collected, usually a bit downward from the fang marks.
3. Apply suction, if necessary, with your mouth. (The venom will not poison your stomach, but you should try to avoid swallowing it.) Suction should be continued for from 30 minutes to one hour.
4. If swelling reaches the constricting band, add another band up about 2 inches higher than the first one.
5. Wash the wound with soap and water; blot it dry.
6. Apply a clean bandage. Ice or cold-water applications may slow absorption of the poison—but do not pack the wound in ice.
7. Get the child to an emergency medical facility as quickly as possible. When there is another adult along or an adolescent who drives, one should drive whatever vehicle is available while the other continues performing the first-aid measures outlined here.

Families who like to hike, camp out, or engage in other outdoor activities during which encounters with poisonous snakes can be anticipated should buy a snakebite first-aid kit, which will contain necessary materials along with instructions for use.

Sneezing

The forceful and spasmodic "ker-chew" by which the body attempts to rid the nose of some irritation. It is a frequent first symptom of the COMMON COLD. Recurrent bouts, often in rapid, machine-gun succession, usually indicate an ALLERGY.

Snoring

Harsh breathing sounds made during sleep. When the mouth is open, the soft palate (spongy tissue toward the back part of the roof of the mouth) vibrates, causing the sound of snoring.

Snoring is usually not of any great medical importance. It may result simply from the nasal congestion that usually accompanies a cold. However, children who habitually breathe through the mouth should be checked by their doctor to see whether they are suffering from enlarged adenoids.

See also: TONSILS AND ADENOIDS.

Soft nails

See NAILS.

Soft spot

See FONTANEL.

Sore throat

Inflammation of the throat, medically known as pharyngitis, is extremely common throughout the childhood years.

Most sore throats occur because of minor viral infections

such as the common cold with nasal congestion, and they usually clear up in a day or two if the child is given plenty of fluids. Allowing a child to use a straw may encourage frequent drinking. A child who can gargle can do so as often as it seems necessary to relieve the pain: saltwater solutions (½ teaspoon salt in 8 ounces of water) or strong tea (either hot or cold) may be used.

However, parents should be alert to the possibility of a streptococcus, or "strep," infection. The only way to make sure a strep infection exists is for the doctor to swab the back of the throat and then culture the specimen to see if it contains strep germs. If it does, then the child is given antibiotics, largely in an effort to prevent RHEUMATIC FEVER. Even if the child feels better and the sore throat goes away, antibiotic therapy should be continued for whatever period the doctor prescribes. Some physicians will, once the therapy is stopped, take another throat culture to make certain the streptococci germs are gone.

Sometimes a child with an inflammation of the thyroid gland may complain of a burning in the neck and throat, but on medical examination the throat appears normal.

When parents are in doubt, or the child seems to have sore throats more often than most children—especially when FEVER is present—the safest choice is to have the child examined by his or her doctor, for sore throat can be a symptom of many disorders.

See also: ALLERGIES, BACTERIAL INFECTIONS, CHICKENPOX, CROUP, HERPANGINA, HERPETIC STOMATITIS, INFECTIOUS MONONUCLEOSIS, MEASLES, RUBELLA, SCARLET FEVER, TONSILLITIS, TONSILS AND ADENOIDS.

Speech

While there are no firm and fast rules about when intelligible speech should be expected, most children are able to speak a few words by the time they are two years old and a complete sentence or two by the time they reach age three. Results of many studies show that when parents consistently talk to their infants using real words and complete sentences rather than baby talk, read to them, and conduct normal conversations in their presence, the babies learn to speak at an earlier age. On the other hand, some perfectly normal, and even exceptionally bright, children seem to prefer not to talk when they are supposed to; frequently these same children begin to speak in complete, well-structured, and cogent sentences when they are three or four years old.

Despite these wide variations in speech acquisition, parents can use the following information as a rough guide to what can usually be expected.

Age	Vocalizations
3–5 weeks	Throaty noises of an indistinct, almost primitive nature
10–12 weeks	Cooing sounds, often in response to adult speech
3–6 months	Babbling is added to the cooing; this may lead to forming the words *mama* or *dada,* and the child may even point to the individual, a proud moment for parents!
10–12 months	Single words, for example, *cat, dog, milk*
2 years	Two-word phrases, for example, *milk gone*
3 years	Three-word sentences, for example, *I want milk*
4 years	Six- or seven-word sentences, for example, *I want milk with chocolate, please*

The great leap in language development occurs from the ages of two to five, with general fluency being achieved by the time the child is six.

Again, parents should be reassured that speech patterns are highly individual; if their child seems slow, they should not worry unduly. Of course, if a two-year-old child cannot communicate even the simplest words, a medical evaluation is in order to make sure the toddler is not suffering from a HEARING LOSS or congenital DEAFNESS.

See also: STUTTERING.

Spider bites

Although most spiders in the United States are venomous and many people are bitten each year, there are only about four deaths during a year.

Of the most dangerous species—the black widow, the brown recluse or violin spider, the jumping spiders, the trap-door spiders, the running spiders, tarantulas, and crab spiders—children are most bothered by the venom of the black widow and the brown recluse.

Signs and symptoms include a skin rash, itching, fever, nausea, vomiting, anxiety, sweating, weakness, and possible breathing difficulties.

Temporary relief of pain can be achieved by placing an ice cube over the bite. No other first-aid measures are of real value, and the child should be taken to a doctor or emergency medical facility at once.

Spinal curvature

Slouching and other signs of poor posture do not cause spinal curvature. In fact, although there is a tendency for the disorder to run in families, doctors can rarely find a specific cause for these curvatures. Apparently a difference in growth rates of the vertebrae (the bones of the spinal column) causes a twisting or bending of the spine.

Kyphosis, an exaggeration of the normal front-to-back curve, is rare in children.

Scoliosis, however, is not at all uncommon. This side-to-side or S-shaped curve seems to affect a number of girls around the time they reach puberty and rapidly grow as adolescents. Some studies show that careful screening may uncover cases in younger children. First signs may be a subtle difference in shoulder height or, when the child is viewed from behind, one side of the back is more prominent than the other.

Most doctors will refer the young person to an orthopedist for an expert opinion. Periodic physical examinations and X rays may be required. In very mild cases special exercises may be recommended. In intermediate cases a brace may be prescribed. These modern braces allow a child to move around and engage in all normal activities, but they certainly cause a lot of emotional turmoil in young adolescents who are just beginning to care about their appearance. Parents and other family members should be prepared to offer considerable support and reassuring understanding.

Only in the most severe cases is surgery recommended, if, for example, there is a danger that chest distortions that might interfere with normal heart and lung function. Prompt professional care stops the progression of the curve and avoids a significant deformity.

Spitting up

The regurgitation of milk drunk by infants. It differs from vomiting in that it is not forceful; fluids tend simply to dribble out of the mouth and onto the chin. It may occur just after a feeding or as long as two hours later, in which case the fluid may be sour, because of the actions of digestive acids on the milk.

As long as the infant is thriving and there is no true vomiting, spitting up is more of a nuisance than a serious problem. Keeping the baby somewhat upright for twenty minutes after each feeding may lessen spitting up. Careful attention should also be paid to the amount of milk given, since overfeeding increases the problem. Parents should also avoid vigorous handling or play right after the baby is fed.

If the spitting up continues to present problems, the child's doctor may recommend a cereal-thickened formula.

Compare PYLORIC STENOSIS.

Squint

See STRABISMUS.

Staggering

See FALLING, MUSCLE WEAKNESS.

Stammering

See STUTTERING.

Staring spells

Brief episodes in which a child seems to lose contact with the surroundings. Most especially in four- to eight-year-old children with active imaginations, daydreaming or boredom can account for such spells. However, recurrent and/or very frequent staring spells may be part of a SEIZURE DISORDER called petit mal syndrome. Therefore, parents should be alert to a possible need for medical evaluation so that any underlying disorder can be treated.

Stealing

Preschool-age children sometimes experiment with stealing, largely because at that stage they often have not developed very clear concepts of what is right and what is wrong. Also, if young children are forced to share even their smallest possessions with other children, they may feel that there is no such thing as private property and everything belongs to everybody.

Parents should calmly but firmly explain to young children that stealing is wrong, and that if it ever occurs again the child will be punished. Effective punishment might consist of temporarily depriving the child of his or her favorite toy or picture book.

Stealing by older children should be considered strong evidence of antisocial behavior. They should be made to return the item, be punished by withholding from their allowance a sum representative of the item stolen, and/or assigned extra duties so that the indebtedness can be worked off.

Parents must also realize that their own infractions, such as tearing up parking tickets, cheating on income taxes, and the like, may lead the child to believe that disobeying rules is not necessarily bad.

However, if cheating is not common behavior in the family and a child continues to steal, he or she should be evaluated by a professional to see if the behavior represents compensation for some real or fancied lack of parental love or neglect by peers. This is especially likely when a child also shows other forms of unacceptable behavior along with emotional difficulties.

Steatorrhea

See MALABSORPTION SYNDROME.

Stiff neck

See NECK STIFFNESS.

Still's disease

See JUVENILE RHEUMATOID ARTHRITIS.

Stings

Of all the venomous insects, bees, wasps, hornets, and yellow jackets inflict stings that cause the greatest number of deaths in children who suffer ANAPHYLACTIC SHOCK, the most serious form of allergic reaction. The child may collapse. Emergency treatment calls for an injection of epinephrine (adrenaline), which is present in some emergency kits, or massive doses of antihistamine if the child is able to swallow. Even if parents administer first aid—and especially when they are *not* able to do so!—seek immediate medical attention for the child. These reactions can be life threatening. Symptoms include wheezing or difficulty in swallowing, clamminess and poor color, or total and immediate collapse. Once the child is known to be this sensitive, parents may wish to discuss the child's undergoing a desensitization procedure. If the parents consent, the doctor administers a series of purified venom extracts, which builds the child's resistance to future stings.

Fortunately most children are not so sensitive to stings. Unless they are stung inside the mouth or on the tongue (another very serious, potentially life-threatening situation that demands immediate medical care), the normal reaction is simply one of pain and swelling at the sting site.

Sometimes the insect leaves its stinger behind, partly embedded in the skin. Parents should remove the stinger as soon as possible. Ideally fine tweezers should be used, but clean fingernails will do. Try to grasp the stinger as close to the skin surface as possible, since squeezing higher up may force any venom still on the stinger into the skin.

Cold compresses may help the discomfort, and a locally applied paste of baking soda mixed with a little water will aid in relieving itching and discomfort. Children's dosages of aspirin-like tablets can also be given.

If increasing pain and redness or swelling develop two or three days afterward, a bacterial infection may have been introduced through the sting hole; the child should be checked by a doctor.

Compare INSECT BITES.

Stomachache

See ABDOMINAL PAIN, INDIGESTION.

Strabismus

A visual disorder, also known as squint or lazy eye, in which the eyes are not directed on the same object at the same time.

Strabismus can occur anytime from birth onward. It may show up before the first birthday if muscle imbalance is the cause, and all during the preschool years.

Parents should understand, however, that a number of infants, particularly up to the age of six months, show what is called pseudostrabismus (false cross-eyes). It is harmless and requires no treatment, but if it continues after the baby is six months old, it should be checked by a doctor to make sure true strabismus is not involved.

In true strabismus, when children look at an object, only one eye is really seeing it. This is a makeshift, automatic device to prevent double vision, which is intolerably confusing. The youngster simply suppresses the second image. Unless treatment is begun early (say, by the age of five or six), there can be considerable loss of vision, even blindness, in the unused eye. Therefore, young children should be given careful eye examinations that do not rely on the youngsters' ability to report what they are seeing.

Convergent strabismus is the name for the cross-eyed condition in which both eyes appear to look toward the nose. The crossing can be more pronounced in one eye than in the other or when the child is looking at a very near or very far object. In another form, both eyes seem to be looking outward. In most instances, however, only one eye is affected.

The treatment for strabismus depends on the nature of the squint. If only one eye has been used, patching the overused eye may correct the situation. Special exercises may be assigned for muscle imbalance. Eye drops and glasses may be prescribed for some deviations that impair vision. Corrective surgery, often done in stages, is generally recommended for children whose cross-eyedness may cause permanent impairment of vision and/or severe emotional problems from realizing that they look odd to other people.

Stranger fear

A behavior in normal infants, characterized by screaming and strong attempts to avoid contact with anyone except parents or daily caretakers.

This phenomenon is caused by the emergence of what psychologists and other professionals call object identity. By the age of two or three months, most infants have a sense of object permanence, the concept that people and other objects continue to exist even when, for the moment, they cannot be seen, touched, or heard. At about six months babies begin to develop the sense of object identity, by which they are able to sense the unique qualities of themselves and others around them. However, they still feel a strong attachment to their mothers, from whom, at an earlier stage, they could not really differentiate themselves as being separate. This growing individualization, combined with a strong tie to their mothers, sometimes causes a discomforting anxiety.

It is at this time that babies who at one point could be left with just about anybody start to protest loudly when left alone with strangers, even grandparents or other relatives and friends they have seen before. By the time the child is about one year old, he or she has learned to discriminate more finely between one person and the next, is more certain that the disappeared mother or other caretaker will return, and is comfortable with an increasing number of different people after a brief period of getting acquainted. Between the ages of one and two, as children acquire more and more autonomy, they are able to tolerate increasingly longer separations from their mother in the company of others. Some children may at that time become a little shy when confronted by people entirely new to them, but this differs from stranger fear and it, too, is a stage that is normally outgrown within a few months.

Strawberry mark

See HEMANGIOMA.

Strep throat

A bacterial infection of the throat, caused by the germ *Streptococcus pyogenes.* If untreated, such an infection could lead to rheumatic fever.

See also: SORE THROAT.

Stuttering

A speech disorder also called stammering, involving speaking with pauses or blocks and/or rapidly repeating syllables or initial sounds.

During the usual period of rapid language development, from the ages of two and five, nearly all children pause, block, and repeat sounds. No one knows exactly why this is so, but an interesting theory has been advanced. It is thought that although young children understand language and may understand rudimentary rules for sentence structure, sometimes of their own making, they simply lack practice in fluent speech. Therefore the natural flow of sentences gets blocked and, in their effort to overcome any lack of clarity, children's speech may become even less fluent.

If parents or older siblings avoid eye contact or overreact by telling the child to think first, speak more slowly, start all over again, and so on, the child may turn this negative reaction inward, heightening self-consciousness about speaking.

Thus family interaction may be a key factor that leads to psychological difficulties that reinforce the problem. In only the rarest of instances is there any neurological component, and there is no evidence that stuttering is hereditary or even that children learn to stutter by imitating poor speech patterns.

If noninterference remains standard, for example, not interrupting or making demands, and if all the family carefully avoids teasing, then the child who stutters for more than a few months during this language-development phase should be taken for experienced professional evaluation. After ruling out hearing loss or deafness, the doctor may recommend the services of a qualified speech therapist.

Even highly verbal, extremely fluent speakers sometimes stutter if they are overly excited or embarrassed. Therefore, temporary spells of such stammering by children should be overlooked.

St. Vitus' dance

See CHOREA.

Sty

A BACTERIAL INFECTION, usually by the staphylococcus or "staph" germ, that causes a small abscess of a gland in the eyelid.

A child may first complain of eye discomfort. Then a small red bump appears along the eyelid, near the base of the lashes. Eventually this infection comes to a head and a small center of yellow pus generally drains of its own accord. If it does not, ask the child's doctor if it should be drained professionally.

Warm compresses offer some relief. Simply dissolve ½ teaspoon salt in 8 ounces of water, and use a folded piece of clean cloth to form a compress that is applied to the child's closed eye for about twenty minutes. Repeat this procedure every hour and a half. An antibiotic ointment or eyedrops may be recommended by the child's doctor.

Even with the best treatment, sties tend to recur; some authorities believe there may be a hereditary basis for them. Sties never suggest a need for eyeglasses.

Sudden infant death syndrome

Commonly known as crib death, the sudden and unexplained death of an apparently healthy infant.

Sudden infant death syndrome (SIDS) is the most common cause of death in babies between the ages of two weeks and one year, peaking at from three to four months of age, and the second most common cause of death among children as a whole (the first is accidents). In the United States it strikes approximately 2 infants out of every 1000 live births, affecting males more often than females and with highest incidence among premature babies.

Although immediate autopsy is generally recommended, usually the results are confusing. In only about 15 percent of the cases are there definitive findings, such as some unsuspected central nervous system abnormality, an overwhelming infection, or an undetected abnormality of the heart or blood vessels. Certain changes in the baby's airway, liver, heart, or nervous system may be observed, but none fully explains the death.

When an infant is at risk after having an unexplained episode of poor color, stillness, and apparent cessation of breathing, or when the family has already suffered a loss from SIDS, a monitoring alarm system for home use might be recommended. In some cases its use has led to a baby's survival. But routine monitoring of every infant is not advised.

A family who has suffered through a crib death needs very special understanding. They tend to have an almost overwhelming sense of guilt, even when they rationally understand that they are not to blame. Some authorities recommend that professionals visit the home to answer questions about autopsy findings, observe the scene of the crib death, offer reassuring support if parents have had to endure the added stress of a police investigation, and counsel parents both in their grief and with respect to having other children.

A family physician, a local social agency, or members of the International Guild for Infant Survival or the National Foundation for Sudden Infant Death Syndrome can be of help.

Suicide

The subject of suicide makes many people extremely uncomfortable, especially when parents must confront the cold fact that suicide is now a leading cause of death in teenagers, rated second and third in some studies. Between 1950 and 1975 the incidence of adolescent suicide tripled, and the rate continues to rise. This is especially significant because a death is generally not listed as suicide unless there is proof of intention to commit suicide, such as prior threats, suicidal gestures, unsuccessful previous attempts, or a note or statement.

Many parents wrongfully assume that their own adolescent problems can be equated with those teenagers face today. With continuing threats of nuclear holocaust, increasing high technology that imposes ever-mounting demands on youngsters trying to make up their minds about what to do with their lives, and widespread turbulence in people's convictions about many traditional values, each new generation faces more complex problems. When this unrest is coupled with the physical and emotional development adolescents face, some of them decide they can no longer cope with life and the only way out is death.

If parents are able to recognize the seriousness of their child's plight and sincerely show loving concern, the adolescent may reach a new level of maturity in which alternatives other than death become more attractive. This is especially true when, after a suicidal gesture, the teenager realizes that he or she need not go to such extremes to get attention and respect. At the same time, parents must know that attention, respect, love, and concern *in advance* do not, unfortunately, always ensure against teenagers attempting suicide.

The old advice about ignoring suicide threats and the old saying that people who talk about committing suicide do not do it are totally wrong. Suicidal talk, let alone suicidal gestures, are serious cries for help. Such youngsters need counseling with a professional who is experienced with such cases and with whom the teenager can develop a viable and trusting relationship. Concurrent family therapy may be advisable, not only as an acknowledgment of the whole family's interest and support and as a means by which the teenager can express his or her feelings in neutral surroundings, but also so that the rest of the family can learn how their own conflicts may be contributing to the child's dilemma. Some restructuring of the home environment may be in order.

School truancy, sleep problems, preoccupation with bodily health, vague physical symptoms (particularly unexplained headache or abdominal pain), depression, emotional withdrawal, weight loss, irritability, addiction to alcohol or drugs, and running away from home are all signs that studies have shown may indicate escape behavior that may lead to suicide.

Parents should heed these kinds of warnings and ask for professional help. Denying the problem won't make it go away, and long-term follow-ups of would-be adolescent suicides show that most become healthy and productive adults.

Unfortunately, there are times that even the strongest efforts fail and determined children succeed in killing themselves. Trying to relive the past and the whole sequence of events is an unavoidable parental reaction. Parents going through this extremely painful period of bereavement should definitely seek professional help and continue with counseling until they have come to terms with the loss and their own guilt feelings.

Sunburn

Redness, tenderness, or blistering of the skin caused by the sun.

Infants and young children are especially susceptible to damage by ultraviolet rays from the sun or from sunlamps. Even older children, especially if they are fair-skinned, should avoid overexposure.

When children are going to be in the sun for a long period of time, say, at the beach, parents should apply sunscreen preparations to the child's skin and provide protective clothing except for the briefest excursions into the water. Even an umbrella or other tentlike covering does not prevent the sun's rays from being reflected from the sand, thus causing more of a burn.

Sunburned children should be given lots of fluids. Aloe-containing lotions may help replace lost moisture. There are many nonprescription burn ointments, the names of which end in *-caine,* that may offer relief from pain. Be cautious about applying them, however, because they may sensitize a child to those medications. The application of cool water compresses, made from either towels or gauze, may be the safest procedure. Once the swelling has subsided, baby lotions or a cream such as Nivea can be applied. Children's doses of aspirin or aspirinlike tablets can also offer some relief.

A fairly bad sunburn may cause nausea, vomiting, fever

and/or chills, and even delirium. Pain increases as the skin reddens and, depending on the extent of skin damage, blisters. If these signs occur, if the burned area is extensive, or if the burn starts to ooze and look infected, take the child to his or her doctor for appropriate medical treatment, for example, cortisone-type medicines.

Sunken chest

A congenital (present-at-birth) deformity in which the breastbone and chest are pushed inward in a funnel-like shape.

It is more common than pigeon chest and is more likely, in moderate or severe cases, to be associated with heart or lung difficulties, in addition to causing the kinds of psychological difficulties associated with any physical disability.

If X-ray examination indicates the need for corrective surgery, it should be done during the child's preschool years, after the age of two. If it is decided not to operate, the child should have frequent checkups to make sure there is no interference with chest-cavity functioning and to make sure there is no further cave-in, which sometimes occurs during adolescence and requires surgery at that time.

Compare PIGEON CHEST.

Sunstroke

An acute medical emergency, usually caused by excessive exposure to direct sunlight. Unlike in heat stroke, the skin is red and dry. The child's body feels hot to the touch, breathing is difficult, and there may be a loss of consciousness.

The first thing to do is call an ambulance or see that the child is immediately driven to an emergency medical facility. While waiting, or while someone else is driving, the sunstroke victim should be made to lie down out of direct sunlight and with the head and shoulders elevated. The child's entire body should be sponged with cool water, and small sips of cool water may be given if he or she is alert.

Compare HEAT STROKE AND HEAT EXHAUSTION.

Sweating

The body's natural means of cooling itself and maintaining a constant temperature.

Many infants sweat heavily not because of any disorder but simply because they are overdressed in hot weather. During summer or in a climate that is customarily warm, most babies are perfectly fine with nothing more than a diaper. If you must dress them up for some special occasion, use lightweight, loose garments, preferably of porous cotton rather than synthetic materials.

Children normally show increased sweating on physical exertion and also at times of emotional stress. Usually the thirst mechanism causes children to drink sufficient fluids to replace any body fluid loss.

Hyperhidrosis (excessive perspiration beyond what either air temperature or exertion should cause) is an essentially harmless disease that cannot be cured but which can be controlled by medications prescribed by the child's doctor. Excessive sweating may cause skin irritations, but the application of astringent-type solutions or powders cuts down on any discomfort. At times an overactive thyroid gland may be associated with excessive perspiration, nervousness, and weight loss; certain congenital (present-at-birth) heart diseases may also cause excessive sweating, but such a condition is normally detected at birth so the child is under treatment for the underlying problem.

Many people tend to forget that it is possible to sweat too little. Children may suffer a HEAT RASH, called prickly heat, when sweat ducts are obstructed. If the child's doctor or the local pharmacist recommends, moist compresses of Burow's solution can be applied each hour for three or four minutes; relief can also be obtained if the child showers frequently in cool showers.

Swelling

See EDEMA.

Swimmer's ear

Technically termed otitis externa, swimmer's ear does not necessarily come from swimming. Moisture in the ear canal causes favorable conditions for it, hence the popular nickname.

The inflammation may start about the same way as when skin is exposed to fungi or certain allergic reactions; then bacterial infection sets in, usually caused by a *Pseudomonas* germ.

Children may complain of pain, itching, swelling, and a possible loss of hearing. A doctor's examination reveals pus in the canal, which may already have started to drain outward from the child's ear.

Treatment consists of a doctor's careful cleansing of the canal and the possible insertion of a cotton wick so that ear drops can reach all the way through the canal. Antibiotics or corticosteroids are usually prescribed for local application, although antibiotics may be given in oral form if the condition is severe. Aspirinlike compounds may be suggested for the relief of pain.

Children who are susceptible to swimmer's ear tend to have recurrent bouts. They should be warned not to use ear plugs, lamb's wool, or alcohol in the ear. Drops prescribed by the doctor should be kept on hand and used before going to bed on any day the ear canal has gotten wet through swimming or even the everyday activities of showering and getting caught in the rain.

Swollen glands

The lymph glands are like docking points along the channels of the lymph system. They filter and collect invading foreign materials like bacteria and viruses, providing a first line of defense against disease.

Lymph glands are found throughout the body—in the neck, under the arms, at the elbows, in the groin, behind the knees, and in internal body cavities. They are named according to their location.

Swollen glands are quite common in children. They can last for weeks or even months, and some children seem to have some slight enlargement almost all the time. If the child is thriving and healthy, there is no need for parental concern.

On the other hand, persistent swelling could possibly indicate some serious disorder such as Hodgkin's disease or the development of a tumor at the site of the gland. If many groups of nodes show enlargement or if paleness, fatigability, weight loss, fever, or a bleeding problem is present, the child should be examined by a doctor to determine if some disorder of blood cells might be present. Other sicknesses such as INFECTIOUS MONONUCLEOSIS may also cause swollen glands. So all in all, it is best that the child be checked, even if just for reassurance that his or her swollen lymph nodes are harmless.

Swollen testicles

Swelling of one or both testicles may be caused by infection or by injury.

Bicycle accidents and other straddling injuries may cause pain and swelling of the testicles. The child should be examined by a doctor to make sure that twisting of the cord is not present, as frequently happens from blunt injuries, which cause excruciating pain and quite evident swelling. If the cord is twisted, emergency surgery is required.

Compare HERNIA, HYDROCELE.

T

Tapeworms

Children become infested with tapeworms just as adults do: by eating contaminated and undercooked beef, pork, or fish. The infestation, called taeniasis, occurs as a result of swallowing an early form of the parasite, which then develops into a mature adult in the small intestine. Tapeworms are among the laziest of parasites. They have no mouth and no digestive system; they survive by attaching themselves to their host and soaking up nourishment through their body walls. Tapeworms are formed by a growing chain of separate segments. They have long, flat bodies that resemble a ribbon, and some species in the human intestine may grow more than nine yards (8 meters) long.

Unless segments of worms are found in the stool, diagnosis may be elusive because mature worms usually cause no serious symptoms. However, the pyschological effect of a child's knowing that worms are in their own intestines can be devastating. Their presence may produce digestive disturbances such as loss of appetite or a tremendous growth in appetite, as well as abdominal pain and diarrhea. Tapeworms are treated by a carefully combined and medically supervised program of diet, drugs, and purges, which cause the head of the tapeworm to release its hold on the intestinal wall. The parasite is eventually passed out in the stools.

Cysticercosis is a condition caused by the eggs of pork tapeworms. Once the eggs hatch in the upper part of the small intestine, they penetrate the mucous walls and are carried to various parts of the body—underlying skin tissue, skeletal muscles, the eye, even the brain. Diagnosis is difficult, and no specific and wholly effective medical treatment exists, apart from controlling the symptoms.

TB

See TUBERCULOSIS.

Teeth grinding

Known as bruxism, grinding of the teeth is usually done during sleep. It can severely damage the gums and supporting bone structures, eventually leading to a need for extensive periodontal work.

Sometimes children grind their teeth as a means of releasing tension caused by anxiety. Parents may notice a clenching of the teeth during the day and a tightening and relaxation of facial muscles as the child clenches and unclenches. At night the clenching may turn to grinding, often making enough noise to awaken parents. Frequently when the source of anxiety is identified and dealt with, the bruxism stops.

At other times teeth grinding can be an almost unconscious effort to relieve a poor bite when the jaws are closed. The child is attempting to create better contact by grinding away bad pressure spots.

In either instance a dentist can fit the child with night guards, removable splints that fit over the tops of the teeth and correct the poor biting pressure. In order to prevent periodontal damage, these night guards should be worn whenever the child goes to bed. The child's doctor may also prescribe mild tranquilizers until the teeth-grinding habit is broken.

Teething

The normal eruption or cutting through the gums of a baby's first set of teeth, called the deciduous or milk teeth.

There is an extremely wide variation in the times at which teething occurs. A few babies are born with one or more front teeth; in other children teeth may erupt as much as six or more months later than the overall average age. Parents should not consider either extreme abnormal. Nor should they use average teething times as a guide to their child's development; professionals do not use it as an index of growth and development, so why should parents?

That much said, however, most parents are interested in *some* guide to teething expectations, so we include the following table with the reminder that it is only a rough guide.

Age in months	Teeth
5–9	two lower front teeth
8–12	four upper front teeth
12–15	two lower (side) front teeth
10–16	four first molars (upper and lower)
16–20	four canines (third teeth from center, upper and lower)
20–30	four second molars (upper and lower, the so-called second-year molars)

Another rough guide is using the child's age in months, subtracting six, and arriving at the *approximate* number of teeth.

Many babies seem to suffer no discomfort while teething. Others become very irritable, drool excessively, and communicate their discomfort by prolonged, almost incessant crying. They are often particularly restless at night, especially when the first four molars, the grinders, erupt.

Babies like to chew on almost anything, so parents can oblige their teething child with a clean washcloth, as the coarseness appears to be soothing, or a frequently washed teething ring, which should ideally not contain fluid, which could be contaminated. Or gently massage the youngster's gums, which provides some direct relief from discomfort and also establishes the close parental contact fretful babies need.

If the baby continues to cry, becomes severely irritable, or shows any signs of fever, take the child to his or her doctor. Teething occurs at a time when an infant's antibody (infection-fighters) level is not at its peak yet, and what is perceived as teething may actually be an illness.

By the time children are about three years old, they should be checked by a dentist and begin various mouth-hygiene rituals. If a baby tooth is accidentally lost before the permanent teeth are coming in, parental first aid may help the dentist save the tooth. If possible, stick the tooth back into its socket and hold it there or have the child hold it in position. Otherwise wrap the tooth in a wet towel or put it into a container of water so that vital tissues are not removed. Then take the child to the dentist *immediately* so that the tooth can be professionally replaced in its socket. Several procedures may be done, such as root canal work and wiring the tooth to secure it in place.

Telescoping of the intestines

See INTUSSUSCEPTION.

Temperature

See BODY TEMPERATURE, FEVER, HYPOTHERMIA.

Temper tantrum

Behavior in which a toddler screams and exhibits purposeless yet quite forceful motor activity. Flailing of the arms, lying on the floor and kicking, and loud screaming are common.

Temper tantrums tend to occur between the ages of two and four, especially during the infamous terrible twos. Embarrassing as these spells may be to parents caught in the middle of a supermarket aisle or on a visit to grandparents, there are explanations for the behavior that may help parents better understand the child's position.

Youngsters of two to four are just beginning to develop a keen awareness of motor activity and how they can display their own prowess at moving about in extreme ways. This coincides with a time during which very few children are not experiencing verbal difficulties—they sense an inferiority at being unable to express themselves in clear language. Finally, few children of this young age group have managed to acquire any capacity for dealing with delayed gratification—they want what they want when they want it.

During the temper tantrum itself, attempts to intervene are almost hopeless. Communication is essentially impossible. If possible, parents should remove the child to a more suitable area until he or she finishes.

The temper tantrum should *never* gain children what they want, or a negative precedent will be set. Both parents should agree on what limits are set for their child, and disciplining measures should be followed to the letter. Physical punishment only backfires to provoke increases in tantrum behavior. Punishment, which should be consistently followed, may consist of confining the child to a safe but solitary area of the house for a short time, temporarily depriving the child of a favorite book or toy, or whatever similar measures fit best with the particular family's life-style, that is, temporarily depriving the child of his or her usual role in the ongoing activities of life in your household.

Although it may not be possible to avoid temper tantrums altogether, parents can do a lot to minimize or shorten them. It is especially important that parents not fly off the handle when something goes wrong. This clues the child that tantrums are an acceptable way to deal with anger or frustration. Parents should not expect too much of a toddler; he or she finds it almost unbearably frustrating to try to sit quietly while adults talk about adult subjects. Whenever appropriate, bring the child into a conversation. Avoiding unnecessary frustration can also help; children are far more prone to throw a temper tantrum when they are overfatigued or hungry.

Children should also be rewarded for good behavior. Verbal praise, a hug, a pat on the back, and smiles are important feedback for the child. Parents should make it clear to the child how well they've behaved and how good behavior is socially acceptable while bad behavior is not.

Usually the temper-tantrum stage passes within a few months. If it persists for a longer period of time, if it seems particularly violent and threatening, if it's indulged in by an older child, or if other signs of emotional disturbance are present, then parents should check with the child's doctor and possibly seek psychological counseling.

Compare BREATH HOLDING.

Terminal illness in children

Coming to terms with the approaching death of one's child is certainly the most difficult task a parent must face. No matter how loving and supportive one's family is, parents may derive more help from consulting with a professional who specializes in this area—a physician or psychologist, a social worker, specially trained members of the clergy, a specialist in the subject of death and dying called a thanatologist, or meeting with a local chapter of one of the organizations formed by parents of fatally ill or deceased children.

Support is of tremendous help as parents try, daily, to lead as normal a life as is possible for the child, offering comfort during painful medical procedures, discussing whatever feelings and fears the child brings up, and trying to balance concern against undue attention that only adds to the child's own anxiety.

By the age of seven or eight children can tell, from the behavior of those around them and from the likely need for frequent and lengthy hospitalizations, that something quite serious is going on. It was once thought that younger children do not have much concern about death and don't really know what it means. That may not be true; even preschool children have some idea of total disappearance, and the fear of going away forever may haunt young terminally ill children, let alone older children and adolescents. Parents who seek professional counseling for themselves are in a better position to deal with the fright and turmoil their fatally ill child may express verbally or behaviorally.

See also: DEATH OF PARENT OR SIBLING.

Testicles, swollen

See SWOLLEN TESTICLES.

Testicular pain

See SWOLLEN TESTICLES.

Tetanus

Tetanus or lockjaw, once a dreaded and frequently fatal childhood disease, is caused by the bacteria *Clostridium tetani,* which live in garden and farm soil, street dust, even in the intestinal contents of humans and animals, where, in expelled feces, they can continue to live for years. The tetanus germs enter the body through a wound. When the wound is extensive, as from a bad cut on metal, or pus-filled, the germs release their toxins, which then circulate through the body. An early sign of tetanus is lockjaw (stiffness of the jaw). Tetanus ultimately affects the nervous system and causes a spasm of the facial muscles. Sometimes this spasm is so severe that it creates a fixed, hideous-looking smile; raised eyebrows; and rigid neck muscles. Abdominal and back muscles may also be affected, sometimes causing the entire back to arch forward, and rigidity of the chest wall may interfere with breathing. Convulsions are possible.

Tetanus can be avoided by the DPT immunization, which parents should make certain their children receive. Most doctors recommend a periodic booster shot every five to ten years, the variation depending on the product used. Successful treatment depends on getting the child to a doctor immediately after any wound is sustained by a dirty implement, tool, or piece of rusty metal, or immediately after an injury has been contaminated by soil or other dirt. The child's medical record should indicate whether a booster injection is necessary. Antibiotics may also be given to kill any bacteria that may have entered the wound.

Thirst, excessive

Active, growing children lose large amounts of water through perspiration. They replace it by consuming what seems to be an extraordinary amount of fluids. Toddlers may seem to do little else but gulp fluids for days at a time; older children and adolescents may seem to strain the household budget by swilling prodigious amounts of their favorite drinks.

In most cases thirst is a normal and natural way for the body to replace lost fluids. However, if the thirst is excessive and the child also urinates quite frequently, a significant disease process may be present, such as DIABETES MELLITUS or a hormonal imbalance. See the child's doctor if nighttime thirst and frequent urination become a problem.

Threadworms

See PINWORMS.

Throat clearing

Nasal drainage that flows toward the back of the throat often causes children to make hacking or snarling noises in an effort to clear the fluid. Occasionally it results from obstructed air flow, as may be the case with enlarged TONSILS AND ADENOIDS. The child should be taken to a doctor so the cause can be determined and treated. An ALLERGY or UPPER RESPIRATORY INFECTION may be at fault in producing chronic throat irritations and increased nasal secretions.

At times throat clearing becomes a habit, one that can become quite annoying. This seemingly minor situation can be difficult to cope with: undue attention may increase the behavior because it gets attention, and ignoring it altogether may increase it in further efforts to gain attention. One approach is simply to explain to the child that the habit is extremely annoying. Suggest that whenever the urge to clear the throat is felt, the child substitute some acceptable and nonobtrusive behavior such as drinking a glass of water. If successful, offer the child praise for his or her willpower and grown-up behavior.

Thrush

Also known as candidiasis or moniliasis, an infection of mucous membranes by a yeastlike organism known as *Candida albicans.*

This yeast can usually be found in moist body tissues in the mouth, digestive tract, nostrils, vagina, and other body passages or cavities, and it generally causes no problem unless it begins to grow or multiply at an unusually rapid rate.

Thrush is not uncommon in children. Diaper rash provides a suitable growth place.

In mouth thrush, white patches appear along the inside of the mouth and on the tongue and in the throat.

Young girls may contract vaginal candidiasis which has nothing to do with having sex, but the risk of yeast growth can be lessened if the child wears loose clothing and cotton panties rather than synthetics, which do not allow for ventilation. In some cases thrush may develop as a side effect of prolonged antibiotic therapy, which kills certain bacteria that normally restrict an overgrowth of various species of fungus.

At the first signs of this FUNGUS INFECTION, the child should be taken to his or her doctor, who most likely will prescribe an antifungal medicine such as nystatin.

See also: YEAST INFECTION.

Thumb sucking

The sucking response is one of an infant's earliest reflexes, present from the moment of birth. The nourishment taken in and the comfort associated with feeding become quickly translated into a means of soothing and relaxation associated with sucking itself. Parents can provide a pacifier to substitute for a thumb or fingers, but the response is the same: sucking.

Parental overconcern about a child's thumb sucking is quite often nothing more than making much ado about nothing. A child normally outgrows this behavior by about the age of five, frequently because playmates tease the child about baby behavior. Generally speaking, this normal rite of passage should be allowed; parents do not really need to interfere, and they should carefully avoid cajoling, teasing, or punishing a preschooler who continues to thumb suck. Neither should parents use severe measures such as painting the thumb with an obnoxious substance or making the child wear mittens. The puckered thumb, the old belief that thumb sucking interferes with language development, and the fear that thumb sucking will cause serious dental or gum problems before the eruption of the permanent teeth are all concerns that parents can safely forget about.

Parents inclined to the dramatic may wish to have a dentist fit the roof of the child's mouth with a training device that prevents the thumb from touching the roof of the mouth, thus discouraging thumb sucking. The real key, however, remains the child's own wish to stop this behavior, and, left to their own devices, most children will do so at a time that is most appropriate for them. Of course, if the behavior persists well into the school years and/or is associated with EMOTIONAL WITHDRAWAL or other behavior problems, parents will need to seek psychological help.

Thyroid disorders

The thyroid gland is located at the base of the neck. It consists of two vertical lobes, one on each side of the trachea (windpipe), connected by a horizontal lobe so that it resembles a fat letter *H.* The thyroid gland regulates the body's metabolism, which is the rate at which the body uses energy. It transforms nutrients and other substances into the various chemicals necessary to maintain life and health.

The thyroid secretes hormones that are necessary for growth and development. When it overproduces hormones or fails to secrete enough, problems develop that require a doctor's evaluation and treatment.

Hyperthyroidism When the thyroid is abnormally overactive and secretes an excess of hormones. Early signs and symptoms include restlessness or nervousness, sweating, rapid heartbeat, and sensitivity to heat. As the disease progresses, the child becomes nervous and jumpy, shows breathlessness, muscle tremors, a staring expression of the eyes, and, despite an increased appetite, loses weight. The disorder more commonly affects school-age children or adolescents, some of whom may show a goiter, which is simply an enlarged thyroid. It occasionally affects newborns, who are extremely irritable and fail to gain weight despite voracious appetites.

Treatment generally consists of an antithyroid drug; the possible use of radioactive iodine, which destroys part of the thyroid, thus reducing hormone output; or an operation in which a section of the thyroid gland is removed.

Hypothyroidism Here the thyroid is sluggish and fails to secrete enough hormones.

Signs and symptoms vary, depending largely on the child's age. Sometimes the thyroid gland does not develop normally during fetal life. Congenital (present-at-birth) hypothyroidism can lead to cretinism if left untreated. An affected baby does not grow normally; has an enlarged tongue, which eventually may stick out from the mouth; a puffy face; and a snub nose. Mental retardation gradually becomes noticeable, since thyroid hormone is necessary for proper development of the brain. Hypothyroidism is correctable by replacing the missing hormone if treatment is begun before much damage has occurred.

In older children and adolescents, signs and symptoms of hypothyroidism include unusual fatigue, weakness, hoarseness, increased sensitivity to cold, and a pronounced loss of energy and drive. If untreated, the young person may develop myxedema, a condition characterized by puffiness of the face and hands, an enlarged tongue that interferes with speech, abnormal weight gain, dry and dull skin and hair, slowed pulse rate, and a general sluggishness of movement.

In almost all cases hypothyroidism can be successfully treated by hormone replacement therapy, which may have to be continued for life. An adequate intake of iodine should also be maintained, to prevent goiter. This can usually be accomplished by using iodized table salt.

Tick bites

Ticks are small blood-sucking insects which live naturally on dogs and rodents (dog tick and deer tick), on the ground, and in wood (wood tick). The bites of these insects can cause disease in humans in one of two ways. Tick paralysis—a progressive loss of strength usually beginning in the legs and spreading upward—is probably caused by a toxic substance released by the insect in the area of the bite. The recently discovered Lyme disease has symptoms of fever and rash and is caused by the bite of deer ticks. The tick is also a transmitter of Rocky Mountain spotted fever—one of the RICKETTSIAL INFECTIONS. This illness is characterized by a very noticeable rash concentrated on the wrists and ankles, high fever, and a very ill appearance.

Preventing contact with ticks is the best method of control. Areas known to have high populations of ticks should be avoided. In warm seasons, parents should inspect outdoor pets every few days to be sure that no ticks have attached. Children, too, should be examined for ticks by a parent each day, as well as being taught to check their skin especially when out camping or playing in infested areas.

The manner of tick removal is extremely important. They *should not* be crushed with the fingers since this may push infecting organisms carried by the tick into the skin. Burning or removing with heated instruments is not advised either since the tick may explode and release infectious particles into the air. The proper method is to coat the tick with alcohol or Vaseline, substances which force the tick to loosen its grip. Then grasp the tick firmly, without crushing, with a pair of tweezers or forceps. Pull for as long as it takes for the insect to let go. If the head breaks off it can be removed using a needle sterilized with flame or alcohol, in the manner one would remove a sliver. If there is any question about a portion of the insect remaining, check with the child's physician. It is best if the tick can be removed within two hours after attachment for there seems to be no disease produced if caught early.

Tics

Nervous habits that usually involve a spasmodic, jerking movement of small groups of muscles. Often facial muscles are involved, as in blinking the eyelids, wrinkling the forehead, grimacing, or twisting the lips, but some children shrug their shoulders or jerk an arm or leg. Sniffing, spitting, coughing, and throat clearing in the absence of clear-cut physical causes may also qualify as tics.

Tics most often develop in the mid-school-age period, around the age of ten, but they can occur in younger and in older children. Tension seems to be the most prominent cause. This may require parents to reexamine day-to-day living patterns in the home; readjust their own expectations (achievement anxiety may lead children to develop tics); and perhaps help the child explore ways in which he or she might profitably cut back on strain-inducing, competitive activities. The child can be reminded gently of the tic when it occurs and how it may be upsetting to people who watch it, but the young person should never be scolded or punished.

Most tics disappear of their own accord as the child outgrows the tension point. Few tics have any neurological basis. However, parents—and the child, too—may want to seek professional help to make sure that a disorder such as TOURETTE'S SYNDROME is not present, as well as for some guidance in sorting out reasons for the tic and how it might be managed.

Tinea

See RINGWORM.

Tingling sensations

Children occasionally complain of a funny feeling or tingling of the face or hands, especially when they are under some emotional stress. If this happens rarely and the spell is brief, parents need not be concerned. Tingling around the mouth and at the fingertips is common during episodes of HYPERVENTILATION.

Abnormal sensations that persist and recur, especially if the child also shows signs of unsteadiness and muscle weakness, should be medically evaluated to be sure no neurological disorder is present.

Tinnitus

The sensation of a buzzing, ringing, or roaring sound in the ear.

It may result from a mild head injury or blow to the ear, from the presence of water or too much wax in the outer canal, or from overexposure to extremely high noise levels.

However, if a child complains repeatedly of hearing abnormal sounds, he or she should be examined by a physician. Tinnitus may be associated with EAR INFECTIONS, damage to nerves supplying the ear, or, on rare occasion, some psychiatric disorder.

Parents need also to be reminded that tinnitus sometimes results from use or overuse of a number of prescription and nonprescription drugs. If this happens, notify the child's doctor immediately so that the dosage can be adjusted or another product can be substituted.

Tiredness

See FATIGABILITY.

Toeing in

Walking with the toes pointed toward the center of the body. It is very common in early childhood, but in most circumstances it is outgrown before the child is of school age.

While the baby is in the uterus, the legs and feet are folded across the lower part of the body. It takes several months for the tendency to this position to change, and it does not happen fully until the infant stands and walks around.

In some cases toeing in may be caused by tibial or femoral torsion, or by a curved or hooked foot. Most cases of tibial torsion (rotation of the shinbone) correct themselves, although severe cases may warrant the use of special night braces. Femoral torsion (rotation of the thigh bone) is also generally outgrown; braces and special shoes do not seem to help.

Metatarsus adductus (a hooked foot) may be corrected by special exercises that press the toes outward. As this condition is often noticed when a baby is only a few weeks old, parents may be instructed by the child's doctor how to perform these stretching exercises on the infant's foot. In severe cases a cast or brace may be applied.

Toeing out

The normal gait of human beings is one in which there is a slight toeing out. Babies do this to a pronounced degree. However, with continued weight bearing, the feet rotate inward until a more usual position is attained.

Concern should arise only if there seems to be no change after a few months, if the deformity is severe enough that a toddler has difficulty walking, or if it seems that the youngster is walking on the inner sides of the feet. Serious, fixed rotations that may require special orthopedic procedures will usually have been noted by a doctor during earlier, routine examinations.

Toenails

See NAILS.

Tongue inflammation

Reddening and soreness of the tongue are uncommon in childhood. When a tongue inflammation does occur, it is generally caused by an infection. SCARLET FEVER, for example, causes a strawberry tongue, named for its appearance. The inflammation goes away when the infection is treated with antibiotic therapy.

On rare occasions medications or vitamin deficiencies can cause an irritated tongue. The so-called geographic tongue, characterized by irregularly formed white patches, has no medical significance.

Tongue-tie

True tongue-tie involves a short attachment between the underside of the tongue and the floor of the mouth; it should not be confused with STUTTERING or stammering. There is rarely enough restriction to cause any difficulty either with feeding or with speech development.

Unless the tip of the tongue curls downward to a marked degree and cannot be extended out to the gums, no treatment is indicated. If a really significant shortening exists, the child's doctor may recommend a plastic-surgery revision rather than just snipping the tissue.

Tonsillitis

An inflammation of the tonsils, caused by a viral or bacterial infection. Infected tonsils appear enlarged and red and may have white or yellow patches on them. The child shows signs of throat pain, difficulty in swallowing, and fever.

Peak incidence tends to occur when children are between two and six years old, and some youngsters may have three or four attacks each year. Once the particular germ has been identified, the child's doctor may prescribe antibiotics. Allowing the child to suck on crushed ice may relieve the pain. In current medical practice removing the tonsils is generally not recommended unless the condition becomes chronic or the enlargement is extreme.

See also: SORE THROAT, TONSILS AND ADENOIDS.

Tonsils and adenoids

The tonsils and adenoids are similar to lymph nodes found throughout the body. They are believed to act as germ traps.

Children's tonsils normally vary in size. They continue to grow until the child is six or seven years old; afterward they gradually diminish in size. In very young children the tonsils often appear so large that they nearly touch. However, unless they are also very red or have white or yellow patches on the surface, they are probably not infected, as in TONSILLITIS.

Adenoids are situated high on the back wall of the pharynx (throat), behind the opening from the nose. Adenoids, too, are most prominent in young children; before adolescence they usually disappear altogether. When children's adenoids become grossly enlarged, they often make it difficult for a child to breathe through the nose. Postnasal drip, coughing, and snoring are frequent results of enlarged adenoids, as is a blockage of the eustachian tubes leading to the ears, which can contribute to ear infections.

Routine removal of the child's tonsils and adenoids is no longer recommended. However, if the tonsils are chronically infected or abscessed, or if the adenoidal enlargement contributes to serious impairments such as chronic ear infections, double removal may be recommended. In the hands of a competent surgeon, the operation is extremely simple and sometimes may be performed as outpatient surgery. Parents should carefully prepare their child by explaining what will be done, how the child might feel afterward (throat irritation is common; sucking on crushed ice may help), and, to the extent the child can understand, why the operation must be done.

Toothache

Pain caused by dental caries (tooth decay) or, in some cases, the formation of an abscess around the base of a tooth.

Pain may not be a prominent feature of the decay process, so regular dental checkups are necessary to make sure that any cavities can be dealt with at an early stage. These checkups are also useful in getting a child accustomed to visiting a dentist *before* he or she is in pain and ripe for emotional trauma that can make going to a dentist a dreaded event. Proper care of baby teeth may also contribute to good alignment of permanent teeth.

Bacteria in the mouth form an invisible coating called plaque that the most zealous tooth-brushing cannot remove. The decay process starts when acid is produced by bacterial action on refined carbohydrates such as sugar and other sweets, as well as other foods. The acid formed in this reaction destroys tooth enamel and eventually produces a cavity that, if untreated by a dentist, spreads to underlying parts of the tooth. The areas between the teeth and the pits and crevices on the biting surfaces of the molars (grinding teeth) are most prone to decay.

The World Health Organization says that fluoridation (the addition of fluoride to drinking water) has been proved an effective deterrent to tooth decay. Communities where water supplies do not contain natural fluoride have found that adding minute amounts of fluoride (about one part fluoride per million parts of water) offers significant improvement in tooth protection. Although excessive fluoridation may cause tooth discoloration, currently recommended amounts seem to pose no problems.

See also: TEETHING.

Tooth discoloration

Many factors can affect the color of teeth. Babies may sprout darkened teeth if the mother was given tetracycline during the second half of her pregnancy. This also occurs when children under the age of eight are given tetracycline.

Once a tooth has lost its nerve and blood-vessel supply, that is, when it is dead, it appears gray. Abnormal calcium metabolism, as in rickets, discolors children's teeth, as does high fever suffered during the time youngsters are forming tooth enamel. Excessive intake of fluoride can cause a mottling or discoloration of tooth enamel, but this should not happen if water-supply fluoridation does not exceed the recommended levels of one part fluoride per million parts of water.

Gross and permanent discoloration of the teeth can pose severe emotional problems for children. Parents may wish to consult with the child's dentist about the possibility of using techniques in which harmless, enamel-colored material is applied for cosmetic purposes.

Tourette's syndrome

This condition, also known as Gilles de la Tourette's disease, named for a turn-of-the century French physician, tends to begin in childhood, lessen during adolescence, then flare again at various periods during adult life.

It is generally assumed to be associated with some disorder of the brain that does not affect intellect, but the exact cause is unknown. Signs and symptoms include TICS (involuntary blinking and muscular twitching) grimaces, general jerking movements of the arms and shoulders, banging of the arms, grunting sounds, barking noises, shouting, and, in about half of those afflicted, compulsive swearing or the use of obscene language.

Control of the symptoms can often be achieved through using the drug haloperidol (Haldol).

Transvestism

Dressing in clothes generally associated with those of the opposite sex.

Until age four or five, cross-dressing may be a normal part of play. A young child may not even recognize that clothing crosses gender lines; it is just fun to dress up differently. This behavior is done openly and without embarrassment. The child should not be criticized, teased, or made fun of. Cross-dressing is usually a phase that passes when other activities come to seem more important.

If cross-dressing occurs much after the age of five or six, it may signal the child's confusion about gender identity. On the other hand, in view of efforts over the past decade and more to foster sexual equality, children's cross-dressing may not have quite the significance it once had. The practice may become far more of a problem for boys than for girls, since society still attaches a great deal more stigma to boys' wearing girls' clothing and assuming feminine mannerisms than vice versa. Parents may be able to help by gently reminding their school-age male child that while it is certainly *his* business if he wants to wear fingernail polish or a skirt, many people, including other children at school, may poke fun at him and say nasty things.

Occasionally when a boy has been separated from his mother, he may cross-dress in a symbolic effort to create contact with the lost parent. Whatever the cause, persistent cross-dressing in school-age children, particularly if the behavior is associated with other signs of emotional problems, warrants professional consultation.

Travel sickness

See MOTION SICKNESS.

Tremors

Involuntary quivering of muscles.

From time to time physiologic tremors may occur in otherwise healthy children, for example, they may begin to shake when they are intensely anxious. Persistent tremors demand prompt medical evaluation because they may indicate an underlying disease or disorder, such as one that affects nerves of muscle groups.

Compare FEVER CONVULSIONS, SEIZURE DISORDERS.

Tuberculosis

An infectious bacterial disease caused by the tubercle bacillus.

There has been a dramatic decline in childhood tuberculosis, often referred to as TB, over the past half-century or more;

there are now probably fewer than 3 new cases each year per every 100,000 children in the United States.

Some newborn babies may contract TB if their mothers have active—unhealed and contagious—pulmonary (lung) tuberculosis. Drug treatment is usually given, although frequent blood, liver, and ear tests are recommended because of some questions concerning their safe use in young babies. Some doctors prefer to use the BCG (Bacillus Calmette-Guèrin) vaccine to prevent TB in high-risk infants, that is, those born to mothers with active tuberculosis.

The widespread use of pasteurized milk and laws that require the testing of cattle have cut down the number of cases of bovine TB. The disease is usually transmitted through contact with a person who has active tuberculosis. Once it is inactive, the disease is no longer contagious.

What is termed primary tuberculosis is the site where the infection is initially located, usually the lung. The infected site heals within a couple of months. Eventually a chest X ray may show nothing more than a small calcified area where the TB node healed. Generally neither the parents nor the child knows TB was ever present, since there are rarely significant symptoms.

At times, however, that area of primary focus breaks down and reinfection occurs. The child or adolescent looks quite ill, and fever, night sweats, difficult breathing, cough, weight loss, and malaise (a generalized feeling of being unwell) are present.

Treatment includes isoniazid (a potent antituberculosis drug), an appropriate antibiotic, and a healthy diet with vitamin supplements. Once the child feels better, resting is no longer considered necessary, nor is the isolation that was once required. After the disease is under control, the child should return to school. If necessary, the child's doctor, who uses periodic X rays to check gradual disappearance of the disease, can explain to school personnel that the condition is no longer contagious.

Two special, but fairly rare, kinds of TB should be mentioned. Miliary tuberculosis occurs when there is a massive invasion of the bloodstream by TB germs. Children affected have ANOREXIA, fail to thrive, and run a fever; medical examination reveals a swollen liver and spleen, and X rays show widespread mottling of the lungs. In tubercular meningitis, the infection spreads to the central nervous system and causes fever, irritability, stiff neck, seizures, and perhaps coma. As a parent might guess, immediate medical treatment is necessary.

Many schools and other facilities give routine screening tests for TB. Small amounts of tuberculin are injected beneath the skin. A positive reaction produces a red area of inflammation, which indicates the child may have had TB in the past. A chest X ray is recommended as follow-up to a positive skin test.

U

Umbilical cord

When the umbilical cord is cut at delivery, a small stump of it is left. Attending personnel generally paint it with a drying, antibacterial dye. It takes about a week to ten days before the cord stump falls off; in some cases this may not occur for three or four weeks. When it falls off, small amounts of oozing and bleeding are normal.

During this healing time parents should apply alcohol to the base of the cord at least twice a day or whenever the baby's diapers are changed. This dabbing with alcohol should be continued for a few days after the cord falls off, then stopped when the area is clean and remains dry.

If there is no sign of infection (such as unusual drainage), nothing more need be done. Large amounts of thick, yellow-colored material, especially if foul-smelling, may indicate a bacterial infection. Redness spreading away from the base of the cord and onto the skin of the abdominal wall signals a spread of infection. Since newborns cannot localize infections very well, that is, infections tend to spread from one locale over larger areas, medical evaluation is needed to see if antibiotics are required.

Sometimes after the cord has fallen off a small red elevation remains on the cord stump, called an umbilical granuloma, representing an area that has not healed completely, and yellow-red drainage may occur. Cauterization performed by a doctor usually allows for rapid healing. In extremely rare circumstances there may be an abnormal connection between the base of the cord and another structure within the abdominal cavity. As a result of this abnormality, large amounts of clear, urinelike fluid may drain from the cord stump. Newborns with this condition should be taken to a doctor as soon as possible.

Underachievement

The failure of a child to perform at a level consistent with his or her abilities.

Parents should be realistic about children's underachievement. It is natural for parents to think that their children are brighter, more creative, more talented, and more motivated than they are. A professor of literature may be baffled when her small daughter shows no more than an average aptitude for talking, reading, and writing. A master mechanic may be dumbfounded when his six-year-old son shows no interest in building a small engine.

When parents are quite sure they have not overestimated their child's abilities—and objective assessment by a professional is the best way to be sure—then parents should look for environmental stresses. The true underachiever is usually angry and frustrated, often because he or she senses an inability to measure up to what is expected. A classic example is that of teachers who overpraise an older sibling, so that the younger child feels inadequate as a student, even when he or she is intrinsically just as bright as the older brother or sister. It is important for the parents and other adults to stop applying undue pressure and begin to praise and reward a child for what he or she *does* do well.

If the problem continues and/or worsens, a medical evaluation is necessary to make sure there is no slowly developing chronic illness or no vision or hearing problem that may be interfering with the child's performance. DEPRESSION also lowers the child's urge to excel, or even to perform at all.

Underweight

Children who are thin are not necessarily ill. During the growing years, a child's weight becomes important only if there is a consistent failure to gain weight or a significant loss of weight.

If the child's level of activity and increase in height are normal, the thin child faces fewer problems with weight control as an adult. Weight-to-height proportions should be kept in mind, especially within the framework of genetic characteristics the child may reasonably be expected to have. However, slavishly following charts of average weight gains anticipated for certain age groups may cause more parental concern than is warranted.

It is extremely unusual for a child to lose weight while growing. The evidence should be documented by at least a couple of weight measurements or, if a child levels off and gains no more weight over a period of several weeks, a doctor should examine the child. Infants may fail to gain if they have PYLORIC STENOSIS or chronic DIARRHEA; adolescents, especially girls, may lose weight with ANOREXIA NERVOSA. Signs and symptoms besides weight loss from these conditions generally cause parents to seek medical help.

Undescended testicle

The failure of one or both of the testes (testicles) to assume their normal location within the scrotal sac.

In fetal life the testicles remain high in the abdomen, being connected to several structures, including the vas deferens, a tube that transports sperm (the male reproductive cells). By the time of birth the testicles usually slip down through a canal in the groin and into the scrotum.

Sometimes this descent does not occur, especially in prematurely born infants, so one or both testes remain in the abdominal cavity. In a condition known as retractile testis, a testis may reach the scrotal sac but then be pulled back up into the abdominal cavity. A doctor can manipulate the gland back down into the scrotal sac without surgery.

Although hormonal treatment has been and sometimes still is used, results have not always been promising. Generally speaking, if both testes remain in the abdominal cavity after puberty, the boy remains sterile regardless of whether or not surgery is performed. The operation shows a good success rate and requires only a brief hospitalization of two or three days.

Upper respiratory infection

An inflammation of structures in the nose and throat areas caused by viral or bacterial infection.

See also: COMMON COLD, NASAL CONGESTION, SORE THROAT.

Urinary tract infection

See CYSTITIS, KIDNEY INFECTIONS AND DISEASES.

Urine and urination

The amount and the color of the child's urine are directly related to the amount and the types of fluids and foods taken in. When they are active, thirsty children take in large amounts of fluids and void a large volume of urine that is very light colored because there is more water than waste products. When less fluids are drunk and a larger amount of waste substances must be removed from the body, this concentration of material results in a dark-color urine.

Variations in color, ranging from barely yellowish through straw-color to amber, are common and normal. Appearance varies, too. At times urine looks cloudy because normal crystals are present. If the urine is allowed to cool and sit, the cloudiness increases.

Children's control over urination comes a little later than their control over bowel movements. Daytime control is usually achieved by the age of three or four years; bedwetting and daytime accidents generally stop by about age five.

Parents generally need not concern themselves about the frequency and appearance of their children's urine unless other symptoms and signs are present. For example, frequency and dilute urine may suggest DIABETES MELLITUS if accompanied by unusually excessive thirst. Painful and frequent urination, BLOOD IN THE URINE, and ABDOMINAL PAIN could signal CYSTITIS. A KIDNEY INFECTION OR DISEASE is likely when these same signs and symptoms are also accompanied by fever or vomiting. An acute inflammation of the kidneys may be present if, in addition to frequent voiding, the urine is obviously bloody or the color of very dark tea. Bloody urine after an injury indicates damage somewhere along the urinary tract. All these symptoms suggest the need for a medical evaluation.

Urticaria

See HIVES.

V

Vacations, parental

Child-rearing is an awesome responsibility, and one from which parents need brief breaks.

Parent-child separation is ill advised only during the baby's second six months. Roughly from the age of six to about ten or twelve months, infants are dealing with a separation anxiety in their new quest for individuation, that is, becoming an individual being, separate from the mother or other primary caretaker. STRANGER FEAR generally appears at this stage.

Older babies, toddlers, and preschool children may benefit from a few days' separation because they learn greater self-sufficiency and begin to gain some appreciation of the fact that security and love do not depend solely on constant contact.

Whenever possible, the vacation should be carefully planned well in advance. Children should be allowed to spend time with the sitter or caretaker a few times so that they become more comfortable with the contact. If the children are going to be staying at another house, visits should be made so that the surroundings become more familiar. A few favorite toys or other possessions should be packed along with clothes when the time comes.

During their absence, phone calls may be more helpful to the parents than to the child. Frequently children fare better than their parents, who are often prone to ruin their well-deserved vacation by constant worry.

Vaccination

Although there are vaccines against many diseases, the term *vaccination* usually applies to immunization against smallpox, an inoculation no longer given to children as a routine precaution.

See also: SMALLPOX.

Vaginal discharge

Newborns sometimes have a mucus-like vaginal discharge that may be tinged with streaks of blood. Once the baby's body is entirely cleared of the mother's estrogen hormones, the condition clears without treatment. A similar discharge often appears about a year before a girl begins to menstruate.

Small or moderate amounts of a white or slightly yellowish vaginal discharge are normal. However, if the discharge is strongly colored; foul-smelling; and if the child complains of itching, pain, or redness around the genitalia, vaginitis (an inflammation of the vagina) is probably present. The premenstrual girl is highly susceptible to vaginal irritations because the vaginal lining is quite thick, protective secretions are not present as they are in an adult, and good hygienic practices are not always followed.

Specific causes of vaginitis in children may include bacteria that have entered from the skin or the anal area. Parents should instruct their little girls to wipe from front to back, not from back to front. Injuries, rectal or urinary problems, the presence of a foreign body as when a pebble is inserted in normal self-exploration, and certain general diseases as diabetes or pinworms may also cause an inflammation.

In adolescence, a heavy, thick, foul-smelling vaginal discharge may indicate the presence of a venereal disease, although parents should not jump to this conclusion until a doctor analyzes the material. A yellow, cheesy discharge may be caused by a yeast infection, which usually has nothing to do with having sex.

While the girl is an infant and young child, the mother can help maintain appropriate hygienic standards by carefully cleaning the child's genital area, blotting it dry, allowing the area to be exposed to warm, dry room air for perhaps twenty minutes, and applying a bland baby oil to the area. Panties should be white, loose-fitting, and made of cotton rather than synthetics, which do not allow for proper ventilation.

See also: YEAST INFECTION.
Compare VAGINITIS.

Vaginal itching

See VAGINITIS.

Vaginitis

Inflammation of the vagina, often accompanied by intense itching. Symptoms may include an increased urge to urinate, pain on urination, and a vaginal discharge that may contain pus or blood and which, in severe cases, is foul-smelling and extremely copious.

In adolescent girls who are sexually active, gonorrhea may be a cause. However, there are many other possible causes: bacterial infection from nonvenereal germs; yeast; protozoal infections such as trichomoniasis; irritation from the insertion of foreign bodies or from chemicals used in douches; infestation with worms; and, although rare, vitamin deficiency. Medical evaluation is necessary to determine the exact cause or causes so that appropriate treatment can be prescribed.

The temporary application of warm, not hot, saltwater (made with 1 teaspoon salt to 1 pint water) gauze dressings may offer some relief from the swelling and itching. Warm tub baths may also help.

Girls should avoid bubble baths, which inflame the area even more, and avoid wearing panties made of synthetic materials that impede ventilation.

See also: VAGINAL DISCHARGE, YEAST INFECTION.

Vertigo

See DIZZINESS.

Viral infections

Any disease or disorder caused by infection with a specific virus.

Viruses are a wide group of microorganisms much smaller than bacteria. Viruses reproduce only within living cells, to which they attach as parasites.

In general, viruses are not affected by antibiotics or other drugs, although antibiotics are sometimes prescribed in an effort to combat a secondary infection superimposed by bacteria. Prevention, however, is possible for viral diseases such as MEASLES and INFLUENZA, for which effective immunization exists.

As yet there is no protection against any of the more than one hundred viruses responsible for the common cold.

Vision

See BLURRED VISION, DIABETES MELLITUS, DOUBLE VISION, FARSIGHTEDNESS, NEARSIGHTEDNESS, STRABISMUS.

Vitamins

A group of highly complex and fragile substances that, in addition to proteins, fats, carbohydrates, and minerals (inorganic elements such as calcium and iron), are essential for normal functioning, growth, and development. Vitamins help regulate metabolic processes so that energy is converted into forms the body can use.

Vitamins are classified into two major groups: the fat-soluble vitamins (A, D, E, and K) and the water-soluble vitamins (all the others). In some cases breast-fed infants do not receive an adequate amount of vitamin D, although they may receive plenty of C if the nursing mother eats lots of fresh fruits and green leafy vegetables and drinks generous quantities of citrus juices. Many doctors recommend liquid forms of supplemental A, C, and D, as well as iron, for all babies.

As for toddlers, older children, and adolescents, professional opinion seems to be divided. Probably the majority of physicians contend that well-balanced diets and the avoidance of too much junk food provide growing children with all their nutritional needs. Some doctors believe that supplementation is wise, especially when parents consider the nutritional value lost in food packaging, preparation, and in busy families the variety of children's meal times, for example, foods kept waiting for various children to return from soccer practice, music lessons, or other activities.

If parents do choose to have their children take supplemental vitamins or vitamins and minerals, they should be sure to follow label instructions carefully. Too much iron may be dangerous, and too-high levels of vitamin A and vitamin D have been linked to certain side effects.

Voice change

In adolescence the voices of both boys and girls change into those of men and women as the larynx (voice box) enlarges and the vocal cords assume adult size, alignment, and tautness.

Customarily, however, people tend to think in terms of the male voice change because of the more pronounced difference, which is caused by gender differences in voice-box and vocal-cord structuring. Cracking and sudden slides from deep bass to high soprano are normal in male adolescents. Parents, as well as siblings and other adults, would do well to ignore these occurrences. The boy should never be teased or imitated, since this could inhibit his speaking and increase adolescent shyness.

See also: LARYNGITIS, HOARSENESS.

Vomiting

Vomiting, usually accompanied by nausea, refers to the expulsion of stomach contents upward and out through the mouth.

Except when a child is semiconscious or unconscious, when vomited material may seep back down into the lungs, vomiting in and of itself is not dangerous. It may accompany minor ailments and upsets that affect the stomach and intestines.

The greatest danger lies in the possibility of DEHYDRATION, a condition in which there is too much loss of body fluids and a salt imbalance occurs.

The length of time before dehydration sets in varies. If either the frequency of urination or level of activity is decreased significantly the child should see a doctor. A good method for evaluating the possibility of danger is to follow these steps: Give the child nothing to eat or drink for a period of one hour after he or she last vomits. Then give the child one ounce of water. Twenty minutes later give two ounces of water and, twenty minutes after that, three ounces. If the child retains the water, proceed with other liquids and watch the level of activity and for urination. If the child vomits during this two-hour interval, call the doctor right away.

Young babies up to about one year can be given one of the balanced electrolyte solutions which are available in drug stores. These provide all the salts in appropriate concentrations for the vomiting infant. After a day or two the regular formula can be used and those solid foods formerly eaten gradually reintroduced.

When the vomiting is over, older babies, as well as children and adolescents, can benefit from drinking heavily diluted syrup drinks; flattened ginger ale or cola; beef or chicken broth; and munching on crushed ice chips or popsicles. Milk and solid foods should be avoided for at least 24 hours—at which time the child can gradually resume a normal diet after starting with refined cereals, cookies, and applesauce but keeping away from raw vegetables for a few days.

While it is true that, per se, vomiting is not serious or dangerous, it frequently indicates the presence of an infection or disease.

Parents should remember that a combination of symptoms can be important. A pain in the right side of the abdomen along with vomiting may mean appendicitis. Vomiting and a stiff neck may mean meningitis. Vomiting may also occur after sharp blows to the head.

Unless parents are reasonably sure that the vomiting is associated with nothing more than stomach upset from overeating, overexertion, or, say, a mild case of influenza, they should check with the child's doctor about the advisability of a physical examination. This precaution is especially important whenever there is blood in the vomitus or if accidental poisoning is suspected.

See also: ABDOMINAL PAIN, APPENDICITIS, COLIC, CYSTIC FIBROSIS, DIARRHEA, GASTROENTERITIS, HERNIA, INTESTINAL OBSTRUCTION, LIVER DISORDERS, MILK ALLERGY, NAUSEA, POISONING.

Vomiting blood

See BLOOD IN THE VOMITUS.

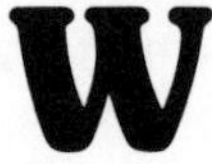

Warts

A viral skin infection that may take as long as six months to develop. One-fourth disappear within six months after they appear; a full two-thirds are gone within two years.

The hands, elbows, fingers, and occasionally the soles of the feet, where they are called plantar warts, are the most commonly affected areas. Warts can be any size, smooth and only slightly raised, or rough and considerably elevated.

Picking at the warts may spread the virus to other areas. Warts need medical treatment only if they are painful, spread rapidly, or enlarge enough to be cosmetically disturbing. They may be painted with special chemicals such as a strong acid, frozen off, or removed surgically.

Wasp stings

See STINGS.

Watering eyes

See EYE DRAINAGE.

Weight gain

After the spurt of growth in infancy and before the spurt common to adolescence, a child may generally be expected to gain approximately seven to ten pounds each year, accounting for the increased size of organs, bones, and other tissues.

The best way of assessing whether children are gaining too much weight is simply by looking at them and carefully seeing if they seem to fit their frames. Obesity in children is rarely the result of some glandular or hormonal problem. There is a strong hereditary influence, but the genetic factor may be overshadowed by the family's eating patterns. If more calories are taken in than are used by life functions and other body activities, the child becomes overweight. If overweight starts during early childhood and becomes a set condition by the age of eleven, the individual is at high risk of being obese for the rest of his or her life.

Treatment is aimed at altering caloric intake while increasing level of activity. Snacks should be eliminated except for raw fruits and vegetables, items such as fruit-juice popsicles, and perhaps some sugarless gum to curb the appetite. Fluid intake should include at least six glasses of water a day; this can be supplemented by skim milk and unsweetened, diet-type drinks. Meals should contain lots of protein in the form of cheese, eggs, meats, and average portions should be served, with no seconds. Desserts are best confined to diet gelatins or fresh fruits.

Diets that cause very rapid weight loss are not advised. Neither should children be given appetite-reducing medications. A physician's evaluation is recommended, and working with a dietician may further stimulate the child's desire to lose weight. Hand-drawn and colored reminders can be posted at particularly crucial spots such as the refrigerator door. The support of self-help groups, for example, summer camps where youngsters go to lose weight, or organizations at which overweight children can freely discuss their problems and successes, have proved valuable in many cases.

Parents, especially, need to cooperate by simply not having high-calorie foods, rich desserts, junk food fillers, and nondiet soft drinks in the house.

Weight loss

See UNDERWEIGHT, ANOREXIA NERVOSA.

Wheezing

A whistling or breathy sound that is usually a sign of some obstruction in the airway to the lungs. As evidence of a breathing difficulty, wheezing may occur in a number of different conditions such as ALLERGY, ECZEMA, CROUP, HAY FEVER, a severe COMMON COLD, and various respiratory disorders.

On some occasions the child wheezes if a foreign body is

lodged in the airway. If the wheezing is not part of an illness already under treatment, prompt medical evaluation should be sought.

Whooping cough

See PERTUSSIS.

Withdrawal, emotional

See EMOTIONAL WITHDRAWAL.

Worms

Although the very idea seems loathsome to most parents, the fact is that children are susceptible to infestation by many types of worms—PINWORMS, TAPEWORMS, and those roundworms that cause a condition called ASCARIASIS.

Signs and symptoms depend on the species of worm involved and on the severity of the infestation. Prolonged discomfort won't occur if the child receives prompt medical attention.

Y

Yeast infection

Candidiasis or moniliasis, the technical terms for yeast infections, are caused by *Candida albicans,* which is responsible for THRUSH and a form of VAGINITIS.

Yeast infection occurs when the organism grows and multiplies at an abnormal rate. This situation may occur as a result of lowered body resistance, such as when bacteria that normally perform protective functions are destroyed by antibiotics given to control some other infection; or when some body change creates a climate more favorable to the growth of the fungus.

Vaginal yeast infections will usually produce a thick, cheesy discharge, which should be carefully cleansed away from the child's genital area. Frequent baths in tepid water and wearing cotton underwear that allows for ventilation will help. However, the only really effective treatment depends on prompt medical evaluation and diagnosis so that an appropriate yeast-fighting drug, such as nystatin, can be prescribed.

See also: FUNGUS INFECTION.

Yellow jacket stings

See STINGS.

YOUR CHILD'S HEALTH RECORDS

Child's Name: Birthdate:

Length at Birth: Hospital:

Weight at Birth: Formula:

GROWTH CHART

Age	Height	Weight

IMMUNIZATIONS

Immunization	Date	Comments
DPT/oral polio		
DPT/oral polio		

DPT/oral polio ____________ ____________

Measles/Mumps/Rubella (MMR) ____________ ____________

DPT/polio booster ____________ ____________

DPT/polio booster ____________ ____________

DT (tetanus toxoid and reduced diphtheria) ____________ ____________

Tetanus booster ____________ ____________

Tetanus booster ____________ ____________

Allergies

Allergic Reactions
to Medications:

PRESCRIPTIONS

Date	Number	Doctor	Prescribed for

ILLNESSES AND INJURIES

Date	Problem	Treatment

HOSPITALIZATIONS

Date	Reason	Treatment

EMERGENCY MEDICAL CARE

Date	Reason	Treatment

DENTAL RECORDS

Date	Reason for Visit	Results

Pediatrician: ____________________(name)
____________________(address)
____
____________________(telephone)

Dentist: ____________________(name)
____________________(address)
____
____________________(telephone)

Directory of Poison Control Centers

Following is a list of state coordinators' offices.

ALABAMA
Department of Public Health — 205/832-3194
Montgomery 36117

ALASKA
Department of Health and Social Services — 907/465-3100
Juneau 99811

ARIZONA
College of Pharmacy — 602/626-6016
University of Arizona — 800/362-0101
Tucson 85724

ARKANSAS
University of Arkansas — 501/661-6161
Medical Science Campus
Little Rock 72201

CALIFORNIA
Department of Health Services — 916/322-4336
Sacramento 95814

COLORADO
Department of Health — 303/320-8476
EMS Division
Denver 80220

CONNECTICUT
University of Connecticut — 203/674-3456
Health Center
Farmington 06032

DELAWARE
Wilmington Medical Center — 302/655-3389
Delaware Division
Wilmington 19801

DISTRICT OF COLUMBIA
Department of Human Services — 202/673-6741
Washington, D.C. 20009 — 202/673-6736

FLORIDA	
Department of Health and Emergency Medical Services Tallahassee 32301	904/487-1566
GEORGIA	
Department of Human Resources Atlanta 30308	404/894-5170
HAWAII	
Department of Health Honolulu 96801	808/531-7776
IDAHO	
Department of Health and Welfare Boise 83701	208/334-2241
ILLINOIS	
Division of Emergency Medical Services and Highway Safety Springfield 62761	217/785-2080
INDIANA	
State Board of Health Indianapolis 46206	317/633-0332
IOWA	
Department of Health Des Moines 50319	515/281-4964
KANSAS	
Department of Health and Environment Topeka 66620	913/862-9360 Ext. 451
KENTUCKY	
Department for Human Resources Frankfort 40601	502/564-3970
LOUISIANA	
Emergency Medical Services of Louisiana Baton Rouge 70801	504/342-2600
MAINE	
Maine Poison Control Center Portland 04102	207/871-2950

MARYLAND
Maryland Poison Information Center — 301/528-7604
University of Maryland
School of Pharmacy
Baltimore 21201

MASSACHUSETTS
Department of Public Health — 617/727-2700
Boston 02111

MICHIGAN
Department of Public Health — 517/373-1406
Lansing 48909

MINNESOTA
State Department of Health — 612/296-5281
Minneapolis 55404

MISSISSIPPI
State Board of Health — 601/354-6660
Jackson 39205

MISSOURI
Missouri Division of Health — 314/751-2713
Jefferson City 65102

MONTANA
Department of Health and Environmental Sciences — 406/449-3895
Montana Poison Control System — 800/525-5042
Cogswell Bldg.
Helena 59620

NEBRASKA
Department of Health — 402/471-2122
Lincoln 68502

NEVADA
Department of Human Resources — 702/885-4750
Carson City 86710

NEW HAMPSHIRE
New Hampshire Poison Center — 603/643-4000
May Hitchcock Hospital
2 Maynard Street
Hanover 03755

NEW JERSEY
Department of Health, Accident Prevention and Poison Control Program — 609/292-5666
Trenton 08625

NEW MEXICO
New Mexico Poison, Drug Information and Medical Crisis Center — 505/843-2551, 800/432-6866
University of New Mexico
Albuquerque 87131

NEW YORK
Department of Health — 518/474-3785
Albany 12237

NORTH CAROLINA
Duke University Medical Center — 919/684-8111
Durham 27710

NORTH DAKOTA
Department of Health — 701/224-2388
Bismarck 58505

OHIO
Department of Health — 614/466-5190
Columbus 43216

OKLAHOMA
Oklahoma Poison Control Center — 405/271-5454
Oklahoma Children's Memorial Hospital — 800/522-4611
P.O. Box 26307
Oklahoma City 73126

OREGON
Oregon Poison Control and Drug Information Center — 503/225-8968
University of Oregon — 800/452-7165
Health Sciences Center
Portland

PENNSYLVANIA
Director, Division of Epidemiology — 717/787-2307
Department of Health
P.O. Box 90
Harrisburg 17108

RHODE ISLAND	
Rhode Island Poison Control Center Rhode Island Hospital 593 Eddy Street Providence 02902	401/277-5727
SOUTH CAROLINA	
Department of Health and Environmental Control Columbia 29201	803/758-5654
SOUTH DAKOTA	
Department of Health Pierre 57501	605/773-3361
TENNESSEE	
Department of Public Health Division of Emergency Services Nashville 37216	615/741-2407
TEXAS	
Department of Health Division of Occupational Health Austin 78756	512/458-7254
UTAH	
Utah Department of Health Division of Family Health Services Salt Lake City 84113	801/533-6161
VERMONT	
Department of Health Burlington 05401	802/862-5701
VIRGINIA	
Bureau of Emergency Medical Services Richmond 23219	804/786-5188
WASHINGTON	
Department of Social and Health Services Seattle 98115	206/522-7478
WEST VIRGINIA	
Department of Health Charleston 25305	304/348-2971

WISCONSIN

Department of Health and Social Services — 608/267-7174
Division of Health
Madison 53701

WYOMING

Office of Emergency Medical Services — 307/777-7955
Department of Health and Social Services
Cheyenne 82001

About the Authors

Edward R. Brace, a Fellow of the American Medical Writers Association, is also author of *Pediatric Guide to Drugs and Vitamins.* During his career as a medical writer, Mr. Brace has contributed to many books as well as serving as medical editor of *Good Housekeeping Family Medical Guide.*

John P. Pacanowski, M.D., is a practicing pediatrician at the Guthrie Clinic in Sayre, Pennsylvania, where he heads the Section of Pediatrics. Dr. Pacanowski received his medical degree from Jefferson Medical College in Philadelphia, Pennsylvania. After completing his pediatric residency at John Hopkins University, he received additional training in adolescent medicine at the University of Maryland. A Fellow of the American Academy of Pediatrics, Dr. Pacanowski is a clinical assistant professor of pediatrics at the State University of New York at Binghamton.